Eye Movements in the Critical Care Setting

Aasef Shaikh • Fajun Wang

Eye Movements in the Critical Care Setting

Springer

Aasef Shaikh
Department of Neurology
Neurological Institute
University Hospitals
Cleveland, OH
USA

Neurology Service
Louis Stokes Cleveland VA
Medical Center
Cleveland, OH
USA

Fajun Wang
Department of Neurology
Neurological Institute
University Hospitals
Cleveland, OH
USA

Neurology Service
Louis Stokes Cleveland VA
Medical Center
Cleveland, OH
USA

ISBN 978-3-030-70220-5 ISBN 978-3-030-70221-2 (eBook)
https://doi.org/10.1007/978-3-030-70221-2

This Springer imprint is published by the registered company Springer Nature Switzerland AG
The registered company address is: Gewerbestrasse 11, 6330 Cham, Switzerland

Preface

Because the eyes are windows to the brain, abnormal eye movements are direct and surrogate markers of brain disease. Eye movements and their disorders are thus powerful tools for localizing brain lesions. With the introduction of advanced neuroimaging, many clinicians today rely less on examining eye movements for localization. In critically ill patients, however, observing spontaneous or reflexive eye movements can still provide important information about the brain.

Nevertheless, eye movements are infrequently utilized in the intensive care unit as objective measures of brain function. This is likely because most critical care providers have little training in neuro-ophthalmology, and neuro-ophthalmologists are rare and practice mainly in the outpatient setting. For these reasons, we set out to create a simple and straightforward guide to eye movements in critically ill patients, primarily for intensivists and other providers who are not experts in the field of neuro-ophthalmology.

How this book came to fruition is worth noting. One of its authors, Dr. Aasef Shaikh, developed an interest in eye movements during his neurology training at University Hospitals Cleveland Medical Center and Case Western Reserve University. His enthusiasm received strong support from his mentor, renowned neuro-intensivist, Dr. Michael De Georgia. The idea of preparing a handbook on eye movements for the critical care setting was Dr. De Georgia's, who envisioned that a didactic text on efferent neuro-ophthalmology in critically ill patients would be of significant value to intensivists. Dr. De Georgia encouraged Dr. Shaikh to write this much-needed book.

A few years later, Shaikh met Dr. Fajun Wang, a neurology resident at the same institution interested in neurocritical care. Dr. Wang became the ideal partner for writing this book; he had an intensivist's mind and a passion for eye movements. Dr. Wang brought limitless enthusiasm and, in collaboration with Dr. Shaikh, helped write this book during his residency. Substantial revisions of the text were accomplished when the world was facing the dreadful COVID-19 pandemic. Our academic passion for writing the textbook was combined with caring for very sick patients in a busy hospital.

We wish to thank our colleagues from the Department of Neurology at University Hospitals Cleveland Medical Center, Louis Stokes Cleveland VA Medical Center, and Case Western Reserve University for their unending support and encouragement. We offer a special thanks to mentors Dr. John Leigh, professor emeritus and former director of Daroff-Dell'Osso Ocular Motility Laboratory, and Dr. Robert Daroff, chair emeritus, for their wisdom and guidance. Finally, we could not have kept up with a busy clinical schedule and an exciting book project without the loving support of our parents and families: Fatema Ghasia, Taahir Shaikh, Zahra Shaikh, and Jiaqi Yu.

Chagrin Falls, OH, USA Aasef Shaikh
Cleveland, OH, USA Fajun Wang

Contents

1 Primer on Examination and Interpretation of Eye Movements in Critically Ill Patients

The goal of this chapter is to provide an overview of eye movement and vestibular examination in relevance to those with critically illness. We will outline the effective ways to examine the eye movements and vestibular function. Our focus is on four aspects of the ocular motor examination; the gaze-holding, saccades, pursuit, and vestibulo-ocular reflex (VOR).

Defining and Differentiating the Disorders of Stable Gaze

The fundamental function, gaze-holding, keeps the eyes steady at the desired location. Although the eyes appear "quiet", the maintenance of the gaze recruits several neural pathways; the failure of these mechanisms lead to unwanted intrusions or drifts.

Nystagmus

Nystagmus is a form of oscillatory eye movement that disrupts the steady gaze-holding. The pathophysiology and phenomenology the nystagmus divides it in jerk nystagmus and pendular nystagmus.

A. Shaikh, F. Wang, *Eye Movements in the Critical Care Setting*,
https://doi.org/10.1007/978-3-030-70221-2_1

Jerk Nystagmus

The jerk nystagmus has a trajectory with a slow component and a rapid correction, giving a "saw tooth" appearance during nystagmography. Typically, the drifts are pathological components of these involuntary eye movements, while the quickphase are the corrective physiological components.

Pendular Nystagmus

The pendular nystagmus, as the name suggests, features eye oscillations with sinusoidal trajectory. The movements of the eyes are like a pendulum of the clock where there are no fast components or the disparity in the velocity of back and forth movements.

Saccadic Intrusions

The saccadic intrusions affect steady gaze, but they are the disorders of the saccade. They come in two types, the square waves and saccadic oscillations.

Square Waves

The square wares are back and forth saccades, typically smaller than 2 degrees, with intervening intersaccadic interval of about 200 ms. On some occasions the square waves occur in form of a single event; while on some occasions the eyes with returning saccades overshoot in the opposite direction followed by the third saccade bringing the gaze back to baseline. Sometimes there is a train of back-to-back square waves, i.e., they appear in "cluster".

Saccadic Oscillations

The saccadic oscillations are also back-to-back saccades, but without intersaccadic interval. In the absence of intersaccadic interval the trajectory appears "sinusoidal" but with very high frequency. Unlike other forms of sinusoidal oscillations, i.e. the pendular nystagmus, the saccadic oscillations suggest instability in the saccade burst generator.

Examination and Interpretation of Common Disorders of Gaze-Holding

Nystagmus

Gaze-Evoked Nystagmus

The gaze-evoked nystagmus is the most common form of nystagmus. The eyes, when in the eccentric orientation, drift towards the center followed by a rapid corrective saccade toward the desired eccentric orientation. For example, during leftward gaze-holding the eyes have rightward drift towards the center followed by leftward correction, hence called "left-beat" nystagmus. The right-beat nystagmus happens when the gaze holding is attempted to the right side. The eye velocity during the pathognomonic slow drifts increases as the desired location of the gaze shifts farther away from the central null position. The gaze-evoked nystagmus is also seen in the vertical direction. The upbeat nystagmus can be present on upward eye orientation, while downbeat on downward gaze holding. The eccentric gaze to one of the corners leads to an oblique trajectory of nystagmus, called "side-pocket nystagmus". The gaze-evoked nystagmus typically suggests cerebellar disorders or central pathology affecting the medial vestibular nucleus or prepositus in the brainstem. In case of gaze-evoked nystagmus, initially, the gaze is stable at null (typically in the central position). In those with the cerebellar etiology of gaze-evoked nystagmus the eyes, upon return from the eccentric gaze orientation, have drifts towards the preceding eccentric orientation. These drifts lead to rebound nystagmus. For example, after rightward gaze-holding that triggers right-beating gaze-evoked nystagmus the eyes returning to the central orientation will have left-beating rebound nystagmus. The Fig. 1.1 depicts a schematic depicting the trend of gaze-evoked nystagmus. The central position with circle depicts the stable eyes, the arrow sizes in the figure depict the intensity of the slow phase velocity. Larger arrow represents higher slow-phase velocity.

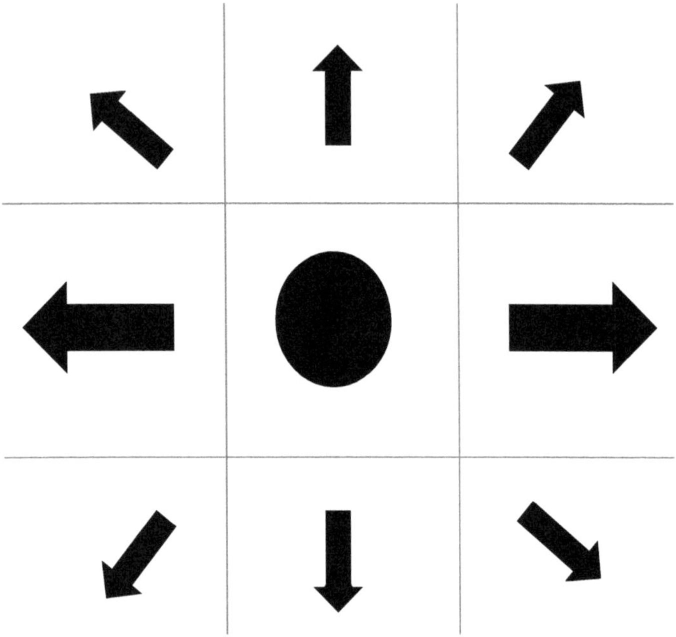

Fig. 1.1 Schematic depicting the ocular trajectory and intensity during gaze-evoked nystagmus. The central position with circle is when the eye velocity is null. The slow-phase eye velocity depicting drifts increase with eccentric eye in orbit orientations. Farther away orientation depicts larger slow-phase eye velocity. The size of arrow depicts larger slow-phase eye velocity. The direction of the arrow depicts the direction of eye trajectory

Downbeat Nystagmus

The downbeat nystagmus is characterized by upward drifts and downward corrective movements. Subtle downbeat nystagmus is often appreciated by watching the movement of the eyelids or eyelashes. The eyes are typically steady in the upward gaze, but it drifts with higher slow phase velocity as the eyes move farther away, i.e., downgaze. In some occasions, rarely, the slow phase velocity of downbeat nystagmus follows the opposite trend. In such rare instances, the slow phase velocity is higher in upgaze, but the eyes are stable in downgaze. Frequently downbeat nystagmus is present as part of gaze-evoked nystagmus, where it changes direction (i.e., converts to upbeat) when the eyes are held in the upward direction in the orbit. Very commonly downbeat nystagmus is most intense when the eyes are oriented in the eccentric horizontal position. Occasionally, the downbeat nystagmus is present after horizontal headshaking, when it is called "perverted" headshaking nystagmus. The perverted headshaking nystagmus suggests cerebellar pathology. Figure 1.2 schematizes the trend of downbeat nystagmus. The stable eye position is illustrated with the circles, while the arrow size depicts the intensity of the slow phase velocity of the nystagmus. The direction of the arrow illustrates the direction of the quick phase.

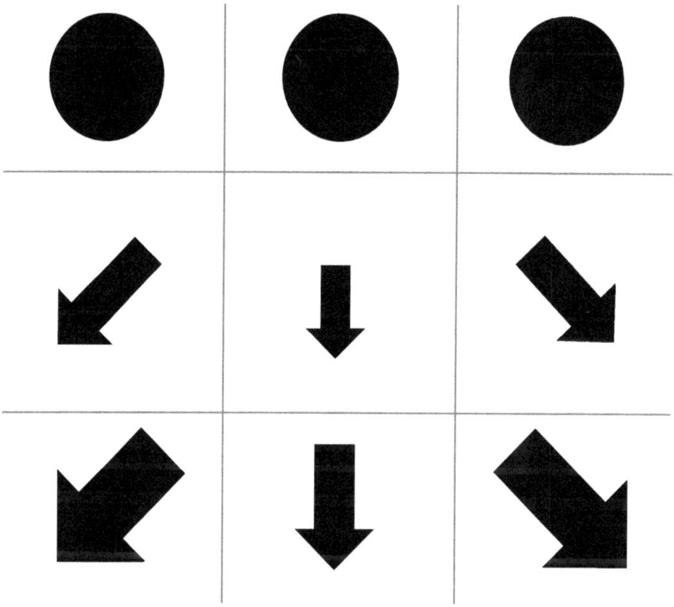

Fig. 1.2 Schematic depicting the ocular trajectory and intensity during downbeat nystagmus. In typical cases of downbeat nystagmus the up-gaze is steady as depicted with a circle. The slow-phase eye velocity depicting drifts increase with downward eye in orbit orientation. Increasingly downward orientation depicts larger slow-phase eye velocity. The size of arrow depicts larger slow-phase eye velocity. The direction of the arrow depicts the direction of eye trajectory

Upbeat Nystagmus

The upbeat nystagmus is rather rare form of vertical nystagmus. In typical forms of upbeat nystagmus, the eyes are relatively stable in downgaze, but the intensity of the nystagmus increases in upgaze. The upbeat nystagmus generally suggests brainstem pathophysiology, but is also seen in patients with cerebellar disorders. The upbeat nystagmus is often seen as part of the gaze-evoked nystagmus when the eyes are directed in eccentric up-gaze. Figure 1.3 schematizes the upbeat nystagmus. The circles depict stable eye position, while the arrow size illustrates the nystagmus

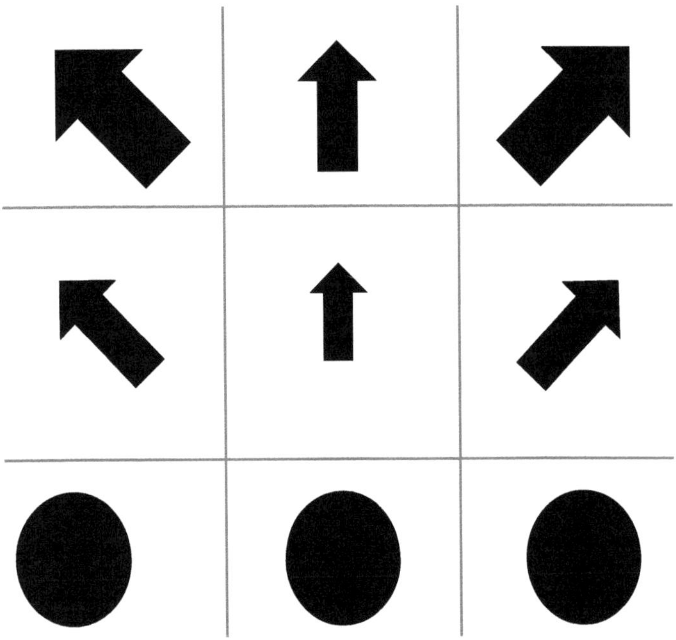

Fig. 1.3 Schematic illustration of the ocular trajectory and intensity during upbeat nystagmus. The downward position with circle is when the eye velocity is null. The slow-phase eye velocity depicting drifts increase with increasing upward eye-in-orbit orientations. The size of arrow depicts larger slow-phase eye velocity. The direction of the arrow depicts the direction of eye trajectory

slow phase velocity. Larger arrow size corresponds with higher slow phase velocity. The quick phase direction is illustrated with the arrow direction.

Torsional Nystagmus

Horizontal and vertical nystagmus is typically symptomatic. The horizontal nystagmus gives sensation of spinning, while vertical nystagmus makes the patients feel as if they are leaning forward or backward. Such mal sensation then leads to unwanted compensation, which is the reason for their fall. Torsional nystagmus is unusual in the sense that it typically does not lead to peculiar symptoms. The torsional nystagmus is characterized by twisting movements of the eyes; hence, typically the foveal image does not shift causing minimal to no retinal image motion. Latter is the reason for lack of perceptual symptoms in those with pure torsional nystagmus. Pure torsional nystagmus, however, is critical to diagnose as it can often lead to the diagnosis of serious movement disorders. One of the classic examples is the syndrome of oculopalatal tremor. This deficit is due to an impairment in the continuity of Guillain-Mollaret triangle and it is frequently accompanied by combination of the torsional nystagmus, palatal tremor, and limb or body ataxia. In other words, it is wise to examine the patient's palate for the oscillations in cases where torsional nystagmus is seen.

Pseudo-Pendular Nystagmus

The syndrome of oculopalatal tremor often have heterogenous form of dysconjugate eye oscillations. They are coarse, neither jerky nor pendular, and disconjugate.

Seesaw Nystagmus

Seesaw nystagmus is an extremely rare form of nystagmus. In this type of nystagmus one eye intorts and moves up, while the other extorts and descends. Such trajectories of eye oscillations lead to an appearance of seesaw in motion, hence the name seesaw nystagmus. Classically describing the lesions in optic chiasm, the seesaw nystagmus can also suggest an impairment in the VOR pathways projecting to the midbrain.

Impaired VOR Matrix

The VOR examination is the critical part of ocular motor and vestibular examination, it is absolutely required in the critical care setting. The VOR is defined as compensatory physiological reflex eye movements accompanying head movements. The direction and speed of eyes are precisely matched with that of head, but they move in the opposite directions. The goal of VOR is to keep the retinal fovea steady on the image of interest, hence preventing an unwanted retinal motion of the stationary images during locomotion. There are three ways to examine the VOR. One is the head impulse test where the head is rapidly moved by the examiner in the horizontal plane and separately in the planes of right anterior/left posterior and left anterior/right posterior semicircular canals. Sinusoidal oscillations of the head are also used to examine the VOR. Head-shaking test is a sensitive way to examine the VOR. The gaze is examined in post head-shaking phase, and normally it should be stable. The post-headshaking nystagmus is induced by shaking the head at high frequency in the horizontal plane as if indicating a "No" response. This test is used to detect the presence of a unilateral loss of vestibular function.

Saccades

The saccades are rapid eye movements made to shift the gaze from one object to the other. The humans make thousands of saccades, voluntarily or involuntarily, each day. The examination of saccades involve assessment of their size, speed, and promptness. Increased or decreased size of saccades, clinically determined by looking for post-saccadic corrections, are called hypermetria and hypometria. The direction of saccades are equally important. The saccades have curved trajectory in those who have atypical forms of parkinsonism. Such saccade characteristic, also known as "round the houses sign", is not only seen in progressive supranuclear palsy, but can be seen in advanced forms of idiopathic

Parkinson's disease. Saccades are normally prompt, but if their latency is increased then it suggests basal ganglionic or cortical dysfunction. The cerebellum has an important role in determining the saccade matrix.

Pursuits

The smooth following eye movements, the pursuits, are examined by asking the patients to follow slowly moving object at bedside. This task requiring coorparation from the patient may or may not be possible in those with critical illness. When abnormal it may suggest number of deficits, interruption of pursuit with intervening saccades are generally seen in patients with cerebellar dysfunction.

Ten Rules of Eye Movement and Vestibular Examination

Rule 1: Be Sure to Have the Preliminaries

It is essential to know that the patient is able to see. The best way to examine the visual acuity is by using the pocket acuity card. The visual acuity may not be feasible to test in every patient that is critically ill, in such cases it may be essential to obtain accurate history assuring there is no baseline visual dysfunction. The fundus examination is necessary to rule out the abnormality affecting the globe; such as cataract or vitreous lesions. It is essential to assure that the lids are not closed due to blepherospasm, hemifacial spasm, or lid apraxia. Latter is not uncommon in those who are critically ill.

Rule 2: Keep the Distance

It is necessary to maintain the distance between the patient and the visual target. We follow the organization illustrated in Fig. 1.4. The

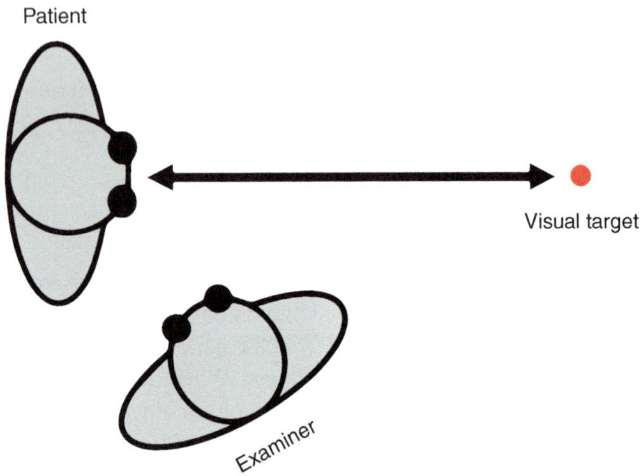

Fig. 1.4 Schematic organization of clinic setting. The position of the patient, examiner and the visual target

distance of about 6–10 feet between the patient and the target is essential to prevent convergence during examination. The convergence can dampen certain types of nystagmus. Keeping the target far away and then bringing the eyes to the hand-held object closer to the subject allows examination of visual angle and depth dependence of the nystagmus. Keeping the target farther away also aids proper examination of the vestibulo-ocular reflex (VOR). The VOR has a strong dependence upon the visual angle, the VOR made to focus gaze on near target has higher gain, that is the eyes move disproportionately more compared to the head movements. It is therefore critical to fixate gaze on the far target while examining the VOR.

Rule 3: Color of the Visual Target Should Be Bright

It is often helpful to use bright visual object while evaluating the eye movements. We use red colored object with a typical tip size of a pen. The red color prevents camouflaging the target with the surrounds, it is easy to see, and can be useful for testing the red saturation.

Rule 4: Check the Alignment of the Eyes

Ocular alignment is not uncommon in those with brainstem or cerebellar strokes or those who are comatose. It is therefore necessary to look for and classify the alignment deficit. One of the reliable ways to examine ocular alignment at bedside includes translucent occlude, however, latter requires adequate alertness of the patient to fixate gaze on the visual target. The translucent occluder allows visualization of both eyes by the examiner, even one behind the occulder; however, the occluder still prevents the vision through the covered eye. Allowing visual fixation leads to re-fixation through the involuntarily turned eye.

Rule 5: Mindful of the Patient's Age and Home Medication Profile

Elderly patients are common in movement disorders. Atrophy, fibrosis, and restricted movements are not uncommon with aging. The typical difficulty in the elderly is to move the eyes up and make full convergence. Isolated, mild upgaze restriction and convergence insufficiency in elderly patient, without any other evidence of parkinsonism, could be simply related to aging. Make sure to keep in mind the patient's home medications while interpreting the ocular motor examination. There are number of medications that cause involuntary eye movements, such as nystagmus. Some medications also affect the dynamics of saccades. Some of the commonly used medications for treatment of movement disorders, such as primidone, can reduce saccade velocity. It is therefore critical to keep in mind whether patient is on one of the saccade slowing agent before interpreting the saccade velocity, especially when it is going to be factored in for diagnoses of some forms of atypical parkinsonism.

Rule 6: Stabilize the Patient's Head

Accurate assessment of the gaze requires proper head stabilization. Even smallest head movement can lead to VOR, and latter can interact with pathological eye oscillations or given impression of having abnormal eye oscillations. Latter are not uncommon in those who have involuntary movement disorders, such as tremor, at baseline.

Rule 7: Pay Attention to the Eyelids

Movement of the eyelids provide important information about the subtle vertical eye movements. The vertical eye movements are yoked with the levator palpabre. As a result upward eye excursion frequently leads to upward eyelid movements. Focus on eyelashes or the lids therefore provides important information on subtle vertical nystagmus, such as downbeat nystagmus.

Rule 8: Use Ophthalmoscope If Needed

The patients may complain of visual deficits, such as blurring or shimmering of vision. Non-specific dizziness and vertigo is also possible without any objective findings on gross ocular motor examination. In such cases, the ophthalmoscopic examination may reveal the mystery. It is important to focus on the optic disc, looking for the involuntary rotations and movements of the disc or surrounding blood vessels. It is not uncommon to find minute disc oscillations, which still can make the patients symptomatic. It is important to know that the direction of the eye movements switch under ophthalmoscopy. The eyeballs rotate on the axis that passes from the middle of it. The optic disc is on the other side of the rotational axis, hence the downward movement of the iris or the front of the rotational axis, for example, is equivalent to upward movement of the optic disc that is behind the rotational axis.

Rule 9: Look at the Bridge of the Nose

It is often difficult to identify subtle disconjugacy between the two eyes. Focusing at the bridge of the patient's nose while looking at the two eyes simultaneously, often makes it easy to appreciate subtle disconjugacy, i.e., seesaw nystagmus, internuclear ophthalmoplegia, or disconjugacy during saccades and pursuits.

Rule 10: Head Impulses Should Be Brief But Fast

Head impulses are important part of the VOR examination. The exam should be performed in all three canal planes; horizontal, right anterior left posterior, and left anterior right posterior. In each plane the head impulses should be fast but with brief excursions. The large excursions of the head impulses will render patients at risk for developing neck pain or even worse sequel such as neck blood vessel dissection.

Approach to Nystagmus

2

The nystagmus is broadly classified in "jerk nystagmus" and "pendular nystagmus". The jerk nystagmus is an involuntary biphasic rhythmic ocular oscillation with alternating slow drifts in one direction and corrective quick phase (the jerks) in the opposite direction. In contrast the pendular nystagmus has slow movements but no corrective jerks, instead sinusoidal to and fro oscillations as the pendulum of the clock. Jerk nystagmus is far more common than the pendular nystagmus, and typically (also throughout this book) the term "nystagmus" is used for jerk nystagmus unless specified as pendular nystagmus.

In jerk nystagmus the slow drifts of the eyes are typically the pathognomonic and they drift the eyes away from the desired gaze orientation. The drifts are generally due to: **(1)** Tonic imbalance in a "slow eye movement" system, such as the vestibular or pursuit systems, or **(2)** due to inability of gaze-holding. The tonic imbalance in the vestibular or pursuit system is typically due to acute asymmetry in the vestibular system, either due to central or peripheral etiologies. The instability in gaze holding typically involves the mechanism called "neural integration" where pulse of neural discharge is mathematically integrated into the step of neural firing rate.

The jerk nystagmus is also classified according to the trajectory of slow phase and according to the conditions under which it occurs. The vertical nystagmus has two types, downbeat nystagmus

A. Shaikh, F. Wang, *Eye Movements in the Critical Care Setting*,
https://doi.org/10.1007/978-3-030-70221-2_2

the second most common form of nystagmus has upward drift followed by downbeat. The upbeat nystagmus has downward drifts and upward beat. Horizontal nystagmus can be evoked by eccentric eye-in-orbit position, when it is called gaze-evoked nystagmus. The gaze-evoked nystagmus is the most common form of nystagmus and typically suggests cerebellar insufficiency. The horizontal nystagmus can be spontaneous without gaze position dependence, it typically suggests peripheral vestibular imbalance. Torsional nystagmus is typically rare if isolated, where the eyes rotate along the front back axis. It is not uncommon to have more than one type of nystagmus coexist, giving them a "mixed" trajectory.

Primary Position Jerk Nystagmus

This form of nystagmus is classified according to the trajectory into downbeat, upbeat, horizontal, torsional or mixed.

Downbeat Nystagmus

The downbeat nystagmus is the most common form of acquired primary position nystagmus and second most common nystagmus after the gaze-evoked nystagmus.

Mechanism

The mechanistic underpinning of the downbeat nystagmus include one of the followings: **(1)** Interruption of the posterior semicircular canal projections responsible for the downward vestibulo-coular reflex (VOR), causing upward drift of the eyes with corrective downward saccades. **(2)** Cerebellar flocculus lesion that impairs the inhibition of the vestibular circuit for the upward eye movements. Latter results in the disinhibition of the upward drifting of the eyes, with corrective downward saccades.

Causes and Management

The downbeat nystagmus is very commonly, about 60% of times, idiopathic. The known causes of downbeat nystagmus include Arnold Chiari malformation, cerebellar degeneration, multiple sclerosis, and vertebrobasilar infarctions. Arnold-Chiari malformation presents with headache and dizziness, which happen insidiously during adulthood. The MRI of the foramen magnum region in a sagittal plane is the investigation of choice. Symptomatic patients benefit from the surgical decompression. Cerebellar degenerations can cause downbeat nystagmus. Episodic ataxia type 2 an is autosomal dominant ataxia which causes downbeat nystagmus. Spinocerebellar ataxia (SCA) type 17 and type 6 are other examples of hereditary causes. Drugs that cause downbeat nystagmus include lithium and anticonvulsants including phenytoin, lamotrigine, and carbamazepine. The downbeat nystagmus can happen even with normal serum levels of drugs. HSV 1 encephalitis can present with altered mental status, aphasia and rarely downbeat nystagmus (cerebellar flocculus affection). The HSV 1 infection also has its hallmark, a lymphocytic predominance in CSF. MRI images show hyperintensity in T2 images in affected areas commonly temporal lobes, the treatment is acyclovir. The stiff person syndrome can present with progressively increasing falls, downbeat nystagmus, stiffness, appendicular and gait ataxia. MRI brain and spine are normal but laboratory investigations reveal increased levels of serum and CSF anti-GAD antibody. The treatment with intravenous immunoglobulin and/or plasma exchange is typically instituted, but outcome to improve downbeat nystagmus remains variable. Other treatment of downbeat nystagmus include clonazepam, levetiracetam, lacosamide, or aminopyridines. The nystagmus resulting from the paraneoplastic syndrome could be reversible if the underlying malignancy is treated without any delay.

Upbeat Nystagmus

The upbeat nystagmus is not as common as the downbeat nystagmus. It is characterized by the downward drift followed by upward quick phase.

Mechanism

The upbeat nystagmus is due to the interruption of the anterior semicircular canal projections, which are responsible for the upward vestibulo-ocular reflex (VOR), causing downward drift of the eyes with corrective upward saccades. Pontine (ventral tegmental tract) or ponto-medullay junction lesions can cause upbeat nystagmus.

Causes and Management

Typical causes of the upbeat nystagmus include vascular (brain stem or cerebellar strokes), cerebellar degeneration, autoimmune conditions such as the syndrome of anti-GAD antibody and demyelination as in multiple sclerosis. Metabolic etiologies such as Wernicke encephalopathy, or toxic levels of anticonvulsants, opiates and insecticides can also cause upbeat nystagmus. Rarely congenital etiology cause upbeat nystagmus and they include anterior visual pathway disease in Leber congential amaurosis. Treatments are often constituted of baclofen, gabapentin, memantine, or aminopyridines. Clonazepam, like other forms of nystagmus, can improve upbeat nystagmus.

Horizontal Nystagmus

The horizontal nystagmus can occur with acquired peripheral or central vestibular lesions. The peripheral vestibular lesions include vestibular neuritis; while central vestibular lesions can cause horizontal nystagmus with gravity or gaze-position dependence.

Periodic Alternating Nystagmus

This is an unusual form of central nystagmus and is considered due to instability in the hypothetical mechanism called the velocity storage. Latter is thought to improve the fidelity of the vestibular ocular reflex and is under feedback control from the cerebellar Purkinje neurons. The patients may complain of episodes of blurry vision or oscillopsia or vertigo. The horizontal nystagmus beats in one direction for approximately 1–2 minutes then stops for 5–10 seconds then beats in the other direction for 1–2 minutes.

Causes and Management

The periodic alternating nystagmus can be seen in neurodegenerative conditions such as ataxia-telangiectasia or SCA6, while it is also present in those with Arnold-Chiari malformation. Acquired lesion of the vestibulocerebellum, the nodulus, is the classic cause of periodic alternating nystagmus. Other causes include tumors, infections, demyelination, autoimmune and drugs. MRI of the brainstem and cerebellum is often critical. If suspected it is necessary to get anti-GAD antibody titer. Routine CSF exam should be considered if infection is suspected. The treatment depends largely on the underlying condition. The baclofen can help with alleviating the nystagmus.

Torsional Nystagmus

The torsional nystagmus typically has a central etiology. It is caused by dysfunction of the vertical semicircular canal inputs form one side. The lesions are commonly at the lateral junction of pons and medulla that involve vestibular nuclei projections. Patients usually have constant nystagmus with oscillopsia. Patients with medullary lesions may have other features of Wallenberg syndrome (lateral medullary syndrome). Patients with pontine lesions may have internuclear ophthalmoplegia (INO) and patients with midbrain lesions develop vertical gaze palsies.

Causes and Management

The torsional nystagmus is commonly caused by infarction and multiple sclerosis. Other causes include tumors, infections, and vascular compression. The diagnostic algorithm includes the brain MRI with high resolution at the posterior fossa. CSF exam is useful if infection is suspected. Trials of memantine and gabapentin has been considered for the treatment of torsional nystagmus, particularly if latter is also a constellation of the syndrome of ocular palatal tremor.

Gaze-Evoked Nystagmus

The gaze-evoked nystagmus is the most common form of nystagmus. Increased tonic contraction of the agonist muscle is needed to oppose the elastic forces that bring the eyes back to the center which results in maintaining an eccentric eye position. Such "step" increase in neuronal firing and muscle contraction correlates with the large "pulse" of force that shifts the eyes to the desired position. Impaired effort to maintain the eyes at the new position resisting the dragging forces leads to gaze-evoked nystagmus. The gaze-evoked nystagmus typically drifts the eyes back to the center, although atypical forms of drift kinematics are also seen in those with gaze-evoked nystagmus.

Mechanism

The impairment in the process called neural integration leads to gaze-evoked nystagmus. Typical source of such deficits are impaired feedback through the cerebellum, vision, or orbital proprioception. The slow drifts of the eyes are towards the center. The drifts are followed by fast "corrective" movements bringing the eyes back to the target. The drifts are minimal at one position "null position". The eye position relative to the null determines the drift velocity.

Drift direction reverses when the eye orientation changes from one side of the null to other.

Causes and Management

The typical cause of gaze-evoked nystagmus is cerebellar lesion, either degenerative, vascular, neoplastic, or immune. Rarely lesions affecting medial vestibular nucleus, a putative site for neural integration, can cause gaze-evoked nystagmus. The MRI brain with focus on the posterior fossa, demyelinating lesions should be considered for the diagnostic algorithm. The treatment generally involves that of the cause. Addressing the offending etiology will mostly result in resolution of nystagmus.

Pendular Nystagmus

The hallmark of pendular nystagmus include sinusoidal oscillations in the 5 Hz frequency range. The oscillations are generally in both horizontal and vertical directions. The vertical and horizontal oscillations have variable phase giving the nystagmus an elliptical shape or oblique trajectory. The key features of the pendular nystagmus is that it transiently halts after eye blinks, or saccades, i.e. the phase reset. The patients typically complain oscillopsia.

Causes and Management

The pendular nystagmus can be congenital or acquired. Pelizaeus Merzbacher disease is an example of inherited disorder leading to pendular nystagmus. The acquired causes of pendular nystagmus include multiple sclerosis, strokes, drug toxicity, and toluene abuse. The brain MRI with focus on the cerebellum, brainstem and sequences that detect demyelination are critical for the diagnosis of pendular nystagmus. Other supporting tests if multiple sclerosis is suspected are CSF examination, VEPs and SSEPs. The treatment of pendular nystagmus largely depends on the underlying cause. Controlled trials show some benefit of memantine and gabapentin. There are anecdotal reports of benefit with clonazepam, perampanel, N-acetylcysteine valproic acid, levetiracetam and lacosamide.

Pendular nystagmus is often associated with head nodding. Typical example of such constellation is spasmus nutans. Those with infantile nystagmus may also present with similar features.

Oculopalatal Myoclonus

Ocular myoclonus can be a mixture of horizontal, vertical and torsional oscillations with a frequency of approximately 2 Hz. They are typically associated with oscillations of the soft palate and sometimes other muscles of branchial origin. The trajectory of the eye oscillations in oculopalatal myoclonus is irregular, quasi-sinusoidal, coarse, and disconjugate. It can present with heterogeneous waveforms and gaze position dependence.

Mechanism

The oculopalatal myoclonus results from damage of the components of the dentate-rubro-olivary circuit, "Guillian Mollaret triangle". The disruption results in denervation of the inferior olive, which subsequently results in pseudohypertrophy. The pseudohypertrophied inferior olive features increased conductance though the connexin gap junctions, causing it to become a generator of synchronized spike trains, which are passed on to the cerebellum. The cerebellar learning processes for timing adjustments then transform into outputs that cause coarse and irregular ocular oscillations.

Cause and Management

The oculopalatal myoclonus is typically a consequence of physical lesion leading to disinhibition of the inferior olive. The cause can be ischemic stroke, rupture of atriovenous malformation, neoplastic, surgical damage, or degenerative etiologies such as progressive ataxia palatal tremor syndrome or multiple system atrophy. Palatal tremor should be distinguished from uvular pulsations that are synchronous with the systolic pulse in patients with aortic regurgitation. The typical treatment includes anticonvulsants such as clonazepam, gabapentin, carbamazepine, perampanel, memantine, valproic acid and agents such as trihexyphenidyl, N-acetylcysteine especially if combined with memantine. Despite many options, the therapeutic success of ocular oscillations in this syndrome is not common.

See-Saw Nystagmus

In this form of ocular oscillation one eye falls and extorts and the other one rises and intorts. The waveform looks pendular. It reaches its maximum on downward gaze. The most common causes are parasellar masses for example pituitary adenoma and craniopharyngioma. Typical treatment include gabapentin, memantine, levetiracetam and clonazepam.

3 Approach to Saccadic Oscillations: Opsoclonus and Ocular Flutter

Definition

Opsoclonus is a form of arrhythmic, chaotic, and rapid multidimensional eye movements. It is not uncommon in critically ill patients who are treated for metabolic, infectious, or autoimmune disorders. Although opsoclonus impairs stable gaze holding, it is a disorder due to abnormal generation of saccades, they appear although not wanted. Opsoclonus is in continuum with the ocular flutter that is a unidirectional, usually horizontal, form of saccade oscillations. The oscillation frequency is the key feature differentiating the opsoclonus/ocular flutter with pendular nystagmus. The latter has a frequency in range of 4–6 Hz while opsoclonus/ocular flutter has a higher frequency, generally in the range of 15–40 Hz. Isolated opsoclonus is possible, but in those with critical illness it is generally associated with myoclonus, ataxia and other behavioral changes. The constellation typically presents subacute but progressive disease process with chronic neurological sequelae in about 50–70% of patients [1]. From the physiological perspective, the opsoclonus and ocular flutter both fall in the category of saccadic oscillations because they are essentially back to back saccades with no intersaccadic interval.

A. Shaikh, F. Wang, *Eye Movements in the Critical Care Setting*,
https://doi.org/10.1007/978-3-030-70221-2_3

Pathophysiological Classification of Saccadic Oscillations

The underlying mechanism of saccadic oscillations allows its classification into two distinct categories: (1) The saccadic oscillation secondary to structural lesions in the central nervous system. (2) The saccadic oscillation due to metabolic, immune, or infectious disorders without any structural deficit. The latter type is relatively more common and frequently postulated to be secondary to disruption to the cell membrane behavior due to disturbance of neurotransmitters, their receptors, or ion channel function. The saccadic oscillations can be idiopathic or can have a familial trait suggesting genetic preponderance.

Saccadic Oscillations Secondary to Structural Deficits

The saccadic oscillations due to structural abnormalities are typically from lesions in the brainstem or cerebellum. Contemporary hypothesis has emphasized the reciprocally innervating circuit of both excitatory and inhibitory burst neurons [2–4] (Fig. 3.1). According to this hypothesis, the structural abnormality in the cerebellum or brainstem leads to hyperactivity in the excitatory burst neurons or inhibition of the omnipause neurons. The hyperexcitability leads to reverberations and consequently saccadic oscillations. For example, injured omnipause neurons and subsequently impaired inhibition to the excitatory burst neurons and/or increased delay in the feedback to the excitatory burst neurons in the saccade feedback can lead to saccadic oscillations [5, 6]. A patient with paraneoplastic saccadic oscillations had a complete loss of the omnipause neurons [7]. On the other hand, cerebellar dysfunction and its influence on the fastigial nucleus disrupts saccade generation [8]. The speculation is that dysfunction of the fastigial nucleus causes delays in the external feedback loop and subsequently leads to the instability of excitatory burst neurons [8–11].

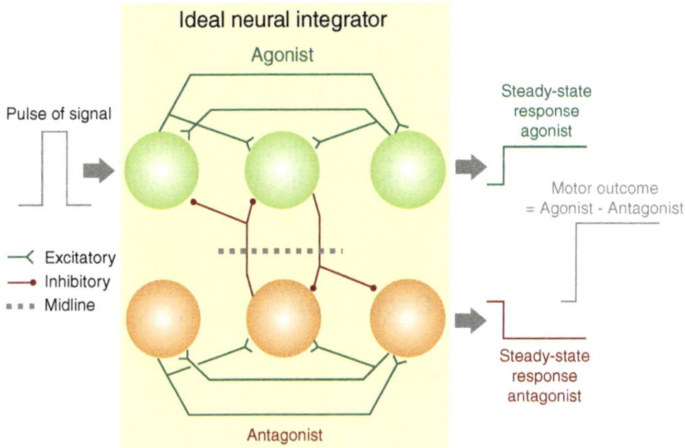

Fig. 3.1 A schematic outlining reciprocally reverberating neural network between excitatory and inhibitory burst neurons. The imbalance in the circuit of reciprocally innervating neurons cause reverberations leading to saccadic oscillations

Saccadic Oscillations in a Structurally Intact Central Nervous System: The Role of Membrane Ion Channels

Saccadic oscillations in otherwise structurally intact central nervous system is by far the most common presentation of such dysfunction critical care unit. Typical etiologies are toxic metabolic encephalopathy, infections, or autoimmune disorders. The contemporary membrane-based theory emphasizes the role of toxins and antibodies in the pathogenesis of saccadic oscillations.

The neuronal circuit responsible for saccadic eye movements is comprised of excitatory and inhibitory burst neurons that reciprocally innervate each other. The reciprocal innervation of the circuit is prone to reverberate but is under constant omnipause neurons inhibition. This arrangement, while enhancing the efficacy of the system assuring high speed eye movements during saccades, however renders the brain the risk of developing oscillations if the fine threshold of stability is crossed [2, 12]. The solution of the risk to oscillations is external inhibition, but it can be compromised too especially when the brain is under metabolic derangement if facing an immune or infectious attack. As a result, it is not uncommon to discover saccadic oscillations in patients who are critically ill due to metabolic, autoimmune or infectious etiologies. In such cases, focus on the inciting etiologies is the most appropriate next step.

Causes of Saccadic Oscillations

Structural Lesions of Brainstem

Structural brainstem lesions can interfere with saccadic burst generation and omnipause neurons-induced suppression of reverberating network. As a result the brainstem lesions can cause opsoclonus. Acute brainstem lesions in critically ill patients are the basis for opsoclonus [13–17].

Hydrocephalus

Increased intracranial pressure can have abnormal stretching and structural interference in midline brainstem structures. Such deficits then can lead to impaired disinhibition of the excitatory burst neurons and consequently cause saccadic oscillations [18].

Multiple Sclerosis and Neurosarcoidosis

Master mimickers of many other neurological diseases, multiple sclerosis and neurosarcoidosis, can potentially affect a number of white matter tracts that could be otherwise instrumental in maintaining balance in saccade generating circuit. One typical way multiple sclerosis can cause opsoclonus is via damage of the feedback loop in saccade generating circuit leading to saccadic oscillations. The other way is through the multiple sclerosis plaque in the connections between the reciprocally innervating burst neurons, or their inhibitory projections from the omnipause neurons [19, 20].

Head Injury

Patients with traumatic brain injury are frequently managed in the intensive care units, especially in the early course. The brain injury affecting the midline fibers via shearing force can lead to structural (often not visible) damage causing saccadic oscillations. It is not uncommon for the traumatic brain injury patients to present for saccadic oscillations on chronic basis [21].

Parainfectious or Viral

Epstein-Barr virus, Coxackie virus, enterovirus, human herpes virus (HHV-6), Influenza, West Nice virus, Varicella, Cytomegalovirus, HIV, Hepatitis C, and recently SARS-CoV2 have all been reported to have opsoclonus [22–30]. Putatively secondary to cross immune reactivity, it can be one of the many grave consequences of viral encephalitis. Latter has to be treated to address the opsoclonus.

Bacterial

Infections caused by mycoplasma pneumoniae, salmonella, streptococcus, and tuberculosis have all been reported to cause opsoclonus [31–34]. Etiology is most likely autoimmune in origin and the treatment is to address the primary infection.

Autoimmune

Syndrome of anti-GAD antibody is known to cause opsoclonus [35]. These patients, typically being followed in the outpatient clinics, often are seen in critical care units for their acute exacerbation requiring plasma exchange. Opsoclonus can also happen in the setting of anti-NMDA encephalitis [36]. In latter, characteristically caused by autoantibodies in patients with ovarian teratoma, the opsoclonus is frequently associated with dystonia, chorea, athetosis, seizure and psychosis. The patients are critically ill requiring early recognition and treatment. Encephalitis and cerebellitis from anti-Ma1 antibody has also been seen in patients with cancers, occasionally seen in the critical care unit if they are severely ill from encephalitis or other comorbidities [37].

Toxic and Metabolic

Opsoclonus is occasionally reported in patients who suffered from the lithium toxicity, overdose with phenytoin, thallium, amitriptyline, poisoning with organophosphates, or abusing cocaine and toluene [38–41]. The patients with nonketotic hyperosmolar coma and Celiac disease can also present with opsoclonus [42, 43].

Summary

In this chapter, we reviewed a special type of eye movement abnormality – opsoclonus. Opsoclonus is a type of chaotic, rapid, multidirectional eye movement. Currently, there are two main proposed pathogenesis mechanisms based on two different categories – opsoclonus with or without structural lesions. In opsoclonus with structural lesion, such lesion generally locates in the brainstem or cerebellum. The presence of structural lesion disrupts the integrity and balance between excitatory and inhibitory burst neurons. And this disruption leads to hyperexcitability of the network. Hence opsoclonus occurs. On the other hand, in patients with intact brainstem structure, cell membrane-based theory was proposed to emphasize the role of toxins and antibodies in the pathogenesis of opsoclonus. Common causes in this group includes autoimmune/paraneoplastic, trauma, infectious, toxic and metabolic.

References

1. Pranzatelli MR, Tate ED, McGee NR. Demographic, clinical, and immunologic features of 389 children with Opsoclonus-myoclonus syndrome: a cross-sectional study. Front Neurol. 2017;8:468.
2. Shaikh AG, Miura K, Optican LM, Ramat S, Leigh RJ, Zee DS. A new familial disease of saccadic oscillations and limb tremor provides clues to mechanisms of common tremor disorders. Brain. 2007;130(Pt 11): 3020–31.
3. Ramat S, Leigh RJ, Zee DS, Shaikh AG, Optican LM. Applying saccade models to account for oscillations. Prog Brain Res. 2008;171:123–30.
4. Shaikh AG, Ramat S, Optican LM, Miura K, Leigh RJ, Zee DS. Saccadic burst cell membrane dysfunction is responsible for saccadic oscillations. J Neuroophthalmol. 2008;28(4):329–36.
5. Zee DS, Robinson DA. A hypothetical explanation of saccadic oscillations. Ann Neurol. 1979;5(5):405–14.
6. Ashe J, Hain TC, Zee DS, Schatz NJ. Microsaccadic flutter. Brain. 1991;114(Pt 1B):461–72.
7. Hormigo A, Dalmau J, Rosenblum MK, River ME, Posner JB. Immunological and pathological study of anti-Ri-associated encephalopathy. Ann Neurol. 1994;36(6):896–902.
8. Wong AM, Musallam S, Tomlinson RD, Shannon P, Sharpe JA. Opsoclonus in three dimensions: oculographic, neuropathologic and modelling correlates. J Neurol Sci. 2001;189(1-2):71–81.
9. Dean P. Modelling the role of the cerebellar fastigial nuclei in producing accurate saccades: the importance of burst timing. Neuroscience. 1995;68(4):1059–77.
10. Lefevre P, Quaia C, Optican LM. Distributed model of control of saccades by superior colliculus and cerebellum. Neural Netw. 1998;11(7-8):1175–90.
11. Optican LM. Sensorimotor transformation for visually guided saccades. Ann N Y Acad Sci. 2005;1039:132–48.
12. Ramat S, Leigh RJ, Zee DS, Optican LM. Ocular oscillations generated by coupling of brainstem excitatory and inhibitory saccadic burst neurons. Exp Brain Res. 2005;160(1):89–106.
13. Keane JR, Devereaux MW. Opsoclonus associated with an intracranial tumor. A clinicopathologic case report. Arch Ophthalmol. 1974;92(5): 443–5.
14. Hattori T, Hirayama K, Imai T, Yamada T, Kojima S. Pontine lesion in opsoclonus-myoclonus syndrome shown by MRI. J Neurol Neurosurg Psychiatry. 1988;51(12):1572–5.
15. Araki K, Ueda Y, Hayafuji M, Takino T. Opsoclonus-myoclonus syndrome with abnormal magnetic resonance imaging and brainstem auditory evoked potentials. Jpn J Med. 1989;28(6):753–6.

16. Schon F, Hodgson TL, Mort D, Kennard C. Ocular flutter associated with a localized lesion in the paramedian pontine reticular formation. Ann Neurol. 2001;50(3):413–6.
17. Tsutsumi T, Murakami M, Kawaishi J, Chida W, Watanabe K. Ocular flutter associated with a lesion of the right upper pontine tegmentum. Auris Nasus Larynx. 2009;36(6):695–7.
18. Shetty T, Rosman NP. Opsoclonus in hydrocephalus. Arch Ophthalmol. 1972;88(6):585–9.
19. Amezcua L, Morrow MJ, Jirawuthiworavong GV. Multiple sclerosis: review of eye movement disorders and update of disease-modifying therapies. Curr Opin Ophthalmol. 2015;26(6):534–9.
20. Gupta P, Shaikh AG. "Leaky" and "unstable" neural integrator can coexist-paradox observed in multiple sclerosis. J Neuroophthalmol. 2020;40(2):226–33.
21. Rizzo JR, Hudson TE, Sequeira AJ, Dai W, Chaudhry Y, Martone J, et al. Eye position-dependent opsoclonus in mild traumatic brain injury. Prog Brain Res. 2019;249:65–78.
22. Verma A, Brozman B. Opsoclonus-myoclonus syndrome following Epstein-Barr virus infection. Neurology. 2002;58(7):1131–2.
23. Kanjanasut N, Phanthumchinda K, Bhidayasiri R. HIV-related opsoclonus-myoclonus-ataxia syndrome: report on two cases. Clin Neurol Neurosurg. 2010;112(7):572–4.
24. Singh D, Sinha M, Kumar R, Shukla R, Ahuja RC. Opsoclonus-myoclonus syndrome caused by varicella-zoster virus. Ann Indian Acad Neurol. 2010;13(3):211–2.
25. Mustafa M, Levin J, Schoberl F, Rominger A. Postinfectious Opsoclonus-myoclonus syndrome in a 41-year-old patient-visualizing hyperactivation in deep cerebellar nuclei by cerebral [(18) F]-FDG- PET. J Neuroimaging. 2015;25(4):683–5.
26. Armangue T, Sabater L, Torres-Vega E, Martinez-Hernandez E, Arino H, Petit-Pedrol M, et al. Clinical and immunological features of Opsoclonus-myoclonus syndrome in the era of neuronal cell surface antibodies. JAMA Neurol. 2016;73(4):417–24.
27. Sahly A, Gauquelin L, Sebire G. Rapid resolution of Enterovirus 71-associated Opsoclonus myoclonus syndrome on intravenous immunoglobulin. Child Neurol Open. 2017;4:2329048X17733215.
28. Radu RA, Terecoasa EO, Ene A, Bajenaru OA, Tiu C. Opsoclonus-myoclonus syndrome associated with West-Nile virus infection: case report and review of the literature. Front Neurol. 2018;9:864.
29. Simon T, Cheuret E, Fiedler L, Mengelle C, Baudou E, Deiva K. Acute transverse myelitis following an opsoclonus-myoclonus syndrome: an unusual presentation. Eur J Paediatr Neurol. 2018;22(5):878–81.
30. Shah PB, Desai SD. Opsoclonus myoclonus ataxia syndrome (OMAS) in the setting of COVID-19 infection. Neurology. 2020;96:33.

31. Ahn AK, Bradley K, Pina-Garza JE. Opsoclonus associated with salmonellosis in a 6-week-old infant. J Child Neurol. 2014;29(7):952–4.
32. Radic B, Cajic I, Petelin Gadze Z, Sulentic V, Nankovic S. A case of adult-onset poststreptococcal opsoclonus-myoclonus syndrome. Acta Neurol Belg. 2018;118(4):541–2.
33. Kim JY, Choi KD, Choi JH, Choi SY. Serial change of opsoclonus associated with Mycoplasma pneumoniae infection. Neurol Sci. 2020;41(6):1589–90.
34. Saini L, Dhawan SR, Madaan P, Suthar R, Saini AG, Sahu JK, et al. Infection-associated Opsoclonus: a retrospective case record analysis and review of literature. J Child Neurol. 2020;35(7):480–4.
35. Shaikh AG, Wilmot G. Opsoclonus in a patient with increased titers of anti-GAD antibody provides proof for the conductance-based model of saccadic oscillations. J Neurol Sci. 2016;362:169–73.
36. Kurian M, Lalive PH, Dalmau JO, Horvath J. Opsoclonus-myoclonus syndrome in anti-N-methyl-D-aspartate receptor encephalitis. Arch Neurol. 2010;67(1):118–21.
37. Brandes L, Mantica M. Paraneoplastic Opsoclonus-Myoclonus syndrome as presenting symptom of primary Gallbladder Adenocarcinoma (2632). AAN Enterprises; 2020.
38. Digre KB. Opsoclonus in adults. Report of three cases and review of the literature. Arch Neurol. 1986;43(11):1165–75.
39. Wong A. An update on opsoclonus. Curr Opin Neurol. 2007;20(1):25–31.
40. Verma R, Kumar S, Biyani S, Singh A. Opsoclonus - Myoclonus syndrome induced by phenytoin intoxication. J Neurosci Rural Pract. 2014;5(Suppl 1):S109–10.
41. Shameer Nijam MN, Thambirajah N, Vithanawasam D, Vithanage K, Liyanage DS, Gooneratne IK, et al. Phencyclidine: a rare cause of saccadic intrusions. Ann Indian Acad Neurol. 2019;22(4):503–5.
42. Matsumura K, Sonoh M, Tamaoka A, Sakuta M. Syndrome of opsoclonus-myoclonus in hyperosmolar nonketotic coma. Ann Neurol. 1985;18(5):623–4.
43. Deconinck N, Scaillon M, Segers V, Groswasser JJ, Dan B. Opsoclonus-myoclonus associated with celiac disease. Pediatr Neurol. 2006;34(4):312–4.

Eye Movements in Patients with Epilepsy

4

It is common for patients with epilepsy to be admitted in the critical care units. On the other hand, it is also not uncommon for the critically ill patients to receive medications with antiepileptic properties. The eye movement abnormalities seen in such patients could be classified in two etiological categories, seen as a side effects of antiepileptics or those accompanying epileptic seizure. This chapter summarizes two subtypes of eye movements.

Antiepileptic Induced Eye Movement Disorders

Antiepileptics (AEDs) stabilize neuronal membrane and connected neuronal networks to suppress unwanted neuronal discharges that cause seizures. Abnormal patterns of voluntary movements can ensue as AEDs modulate neural network properties. The abnormal movements are frequently observed in those patients who are on central nervous system suppressants, such as those admitted to the critical care units. In this chapter we will review the eye movement abnormalities cause by common AEDs. We will discuss basic organization of the neural circuits and how the circuits are modulated by the given AED to cause abnormal eye movements.

The main structures involved in AED-induced abnormal eye movements include the horizontal and vertical neural integrator,

A. Shaikh, F. Wang, *Eye Movements in the Critical Care Setting*,
https://doi.org/10.1007/978-3-030-70221-2_4

pursuit and saccades matrix. The role of the neural integrator is to maintain the position of the eyes by converting the eye velocity to position. The horizontal neural integrator consists of the medial vestibular nucleus and nucleus prepositus hypoglossi in the caudal pons and the rostral medulla while the vertical neural integrator is comprised of the interstitial nucleus of Cajal and the rostral interstitial medial longitudinal fasciculus in the rostral midbrain (Fig. 4.1). The structures comprising neural integrators operate under feedback modulation from the vestibulocerebellum [1]. AEDs can directly affect the function of saccade (pulse) generators

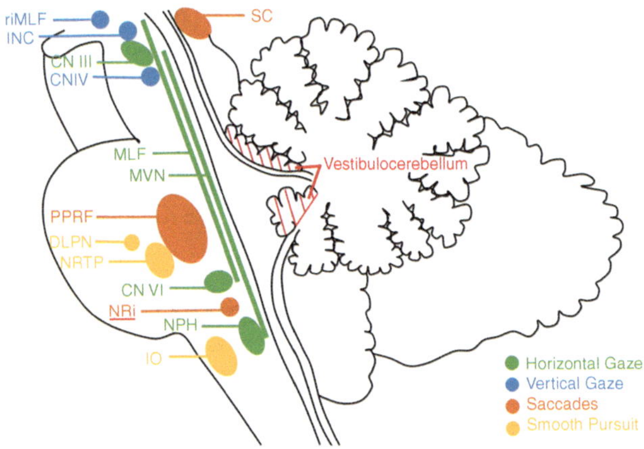

Fig. 4.1 Neuroanatomical Networks: Horizontal gaze network (red): includes Oculomotor nucleus (CN III), Medial Longitudinal Fasciculus (MLF), Medial Vestibular Nucleus (MVN), Abducens Nucleus (CN VI), Nucleus Prepositus Hypoglossi (NPH) and fined-tuned by the vestibulocerebellum. Vertical gaze network (blue): includes rostral interstitial Medial Longitudinal Fasciculus (riMLF), Interstitial Nucleus of Cajal (INC), Trochlear nucleus (CN IV and fine-tuned by the vestibulocerebellum. Saccade network (green): includes Paramedian Pontine Reticular Formation (PPFR), Nucleus Raphe interpositus (NRi); of note burst neurons for vertical and torsional saccades lie within the rostral interstitial medial longitudinal fasciculus (riMLF, labeled in blue). Smooth pursuit network (orange): Dorsolateral Pontine Nucleus (DLPN), Nucleus Reticularis Tegmenti Pontis (NRTP), Inferior Olive (IO), vestibulocerebellum. Vestibulocerebellum is comprised of the flocculus and nodulus, known as the flocculonodular lobe. (Reproduced with permission from Shaikh and Ghasia [52])

or modulate the feedback to the integrator. The impairment in the circuit generating the pulse (i.e., saccade) or converting into step (i.e., steady gaze holding) then leads to different eye movement abnormalities.

Sodium Valproate

Sodium valproate modulates neural excitability by two mechanisms, (1) by blocking the voltage-gated sodium channels; and (2) by increasing the levels of inhibitory neurotransmitter gamma-aminobutryic acid (GABA). The sodium valproate increases the levels of GABA by two putative mechanisms. (1) By inhibiting the GABA degradative enzymes, such as GABA transaminase and succinate-semialdehyde dehydrogenase. (2) By inhibiting the GABA reuptake. All of the sodium valproate induced interventions can also interfere gaze-holding mechanism. The gaze-evoked nystagmus is a common eye movement abnormality in those who are exposed to sodium valproate. Vertical gaze palsy is also possible side effect.

Gaze-Evoked Nystagmus (GEN)

GEN occurs when the patients attempt to maintain the eyes in the eccentric position. The eccentrically located eyes drift towards center followed by a corrective saccade bringing the eyes towards the desired orientation. Impaired neural integrator function has a fundamental role in the pathophysiology of the GEN. The horizontal neural integrator resides in the nucleus prepositus hypoglossi (NPH) and the medial vestibular nucleus. The vertical and torsional neural integrator is in the interstitial nucleus of Cajal, within the midbrain. AED induced abnormality in the function of these integrators then cause GEN [2]. Effects of sodium valproate on neural integrator is one of the main putative mechanisms for generation of gaze-evoked nystagmus. Sodium valproate is known to supporess the firing of the neural integrator network, depressing its ability to effectively transform velocity to position. This phenomenon, a "leaky" neural integration, causes the eyes to drift while attempting to fixate in an eccentric location. Then a corrective saccade is then made to attempt gaze at the eccentric position. This cycle then repeats causing GEN [3, 4].

The brainstem neural integrators are modulated by the cerebellum, particularly the flocculus and paraflocculus Purkinje neurons. The Purkinje neurons, via their inhibitory GABA mediated projections modulate the brainstem neural integrators [1]. The sodium valproate causes dysfunction of the cerebellar Purkinje neurons; with prolonged use, it causes the cerebellar atrophy [5]. Lack of optimized Purkinje neuron function results in deficient feedback to the neural integrators, hence the gaze evoked nystagmus [6].

Vertical Gaze Palsy

Sodium valproate's effect on GABA explains selective vertical gaze palsy seen in those with sodium valproate toxicity. Vertical gaze control centers are in the midbrain; the rostral interstitial medial longitudinal fasciculus (riMLF) and the interstitial nucleus of Cajal (INC). Particularly, the INC has abundant GABAergic neurons. Studies in the macaques discovered GABAergic projections from the INC to the contralateral superior oblique and inferior rectus motoneurons. During upward eye movements, these commissural GABAergic projections inhibit the superior oblique and inferior rectus motoneurons and premotor downward burst-tonic neurons [7]. Toxic levels or basline high concentrations of sodium valproate lead to excessive GABA transaminase inhibition hence reduced neurotransmitter degradation. Subsequently there can be elevated levels of GABA, deactivating the vertical burst neurons producing a selective vertical gaze palsy [8].

Phenytoin/Fosphenytoin

Phenytoin blocks voltage-gated sodium channel and preferentially inactivates its fast-inactive state. The consequence of phenytoin blockade is blockade of high frequency firing of action potentials. Various eye movement abnormalities are reported with the phenytoin and fosphenytoin, however, they do not correlate with the serum levels of phenytoin. The characteristic eye movement abnormalities include gaze-evoked nystagmus, impaired smooth pursuit, impaired VOR suppression, downbeat nystagmus, periodic alternating nystagmus, and pendular nystagmus [9].

Gaze-Evoked Nystagmus

The gaze-evoked nystagmus secondary to phenytoin is due to leaky neural integrator. The mechanism is same as one outlined in the section of sodium valproate. Phenytoin also impairs the central vestibular and cerebellar connections required by the neural integrator. Such pharmacologic impairment of the neural integrator manifests clinically as a gaze-evoked nystagmus and ataxia [9].

Smooth Pursuit

Smooth pursuit are slow tracking of the eyes to keep a moving target on the fovea. The cerebral cortical areas concerned with the visual motion are relayed to the brainstem gaze-holding network which integrates the eye and head-velocity signals, vestibular, and pursuit eye movements into eye position commands. In addition to brainstem networks, the cerebellum also provides information regarding the initiation and programming of the pursuit eye movements. The three components of the cerebellum involved in smooth pursuit are the vestibulocerebellum, dorsal vermis and its projections to the fastigial nucleus, and the ansiform lobule (VII) of the cerebellar hemisphere. Pharmacological inactivation of the vestibulocerebellum in the macaques substantially impairs smooth pursuit and VOR cancellation [10]. The mechanism in which phenytoin impairs smooth pursuit is likely due to its disrupting effects on the vestibulocerebellum.

Vestibulo-Ocular Reflex Suppression

The vestibulo-ocular reflex (VOR) maintains gaze on stationary object during locomotion. Eye movements are generated with same velocity (as head movement) but in the opposite direction, with a goal to maintain steady vision. Smooth pursuit is used to track moving objects while the head is stationary. An instance where the VOR and smooth pursuit systems come into conflict is when the head is moving with a moving target. Here the VOR drives the eyes in the opposite direction while the pursuit system attempts to overcome this by driving the eyes with the target. This mechanism to overcome the VOR is termed VOR suppression.

Impairments in both smooth pursuit and VOR suppression is seen with phenytoin. It may be related to the drug's effects on the cerebellar Purkinje cells and impairing the functions of the vestibulocerebellum. The abnormalities in the smooth pursuit and VOR suppression can be seen even in patients who do not have any clinical or biochemical evidence of AED toxicity. This has been observed in patients receiving phenytoin or phenobarbital and marked improvements are seen after discontinuation of these AEDs [11].

Downbeat Nystagmus

Downbeat nystagmus results from a defective vertical gaze holding causing a pathologic updrift of the eyes and a corrective downward saccade. The presence of downbeat nystagmus seen with phenytoin is likely related to its effects on the vestibulocerebellum [12]. There is a well-known physiological asymmetry in the upward-downward signal driving the vertical pursuit. Such asymmetry in the signal is to compensate for the downward gravity-driven bias. Moreover, the flocculus and para-flocculus Purkinje cells inhibit the vestibular nuclei that receive input from the anterior semicircular canals. Loss of Purkinje inhibition to the vestibular neurons sets free the anterior semicircular canal input. As a result the eyes drift upward followed by a corrective downward saccade leading to downbeat nystagmus.

Periodic Alternating Nystagmus (PAN)

PAN is characterized as spontaneous horizontal nystagmus in the primary gaze, and characteristically reverses its direction approximately every 2 minutes. PAN can be acquired from disruption of nodulus and uvula. These cerebellar structures play a role in the time constant of rotational velocity storage. Pharmacological evidence suggests that the nodulus and uvula maintain inhibitory control on the vestibular rotational responses. Dysfunction of nodulus and uvula can result in an oscillatory shifting of the null point leading to PAN [13]. Phenytoin by disrupting the normal inhibitory control of nodulus and uvula on the rotational vestibular inputs precipitates PAN [14, 15].

Pendular Nystagmus

Pendular nystagmus when acquired is a type of ocular oscillation which often cause continuous oscillopsia. There are typically horizontal, vertical, and torsional components. Depending on whether the horizontal and vertical oscillatory components are in phase or out of phase, the resultant trajectories can either be oblique, elliptical, or circular. The oscillations of each eye can be conjugate or disconjugate. The etiology for acquired pendular nystagmus lies within the neural substrates for gaze holding, the neural integrator. The instability in the network comprising the neural integrator leads to the pendular nystagmus. The phenytoin slows down neural conduction. Such delay in the feedback between the cerebellum and the neural integrator can cause instability. The delayed feedback from slowed neural conduction will disrupt gaze holding due to errors in computation from the integrator. This erroneous eye positioning for gaze holding can then manifest as pendular nystagmus. The instability of the neural integrator from pharmacologically suppressed neural conduction is the likely etiology of phenytoin induced pendular nystagmus [16].

Carbamazepine

Carbamazepine preferentially binds to the voltage-gated sodium channels in their inactive state. The medication prevents repetitive and sustained neuronal depolarization as the anticonvulsant efficacy is due to the inhibition of the sodium channel activity.

Impairments of the eye movements associated with the carbamazepine include gaze-evoked nystagmus, slowing of saccade velocity, impaired smooth pursuit, downbeat nystagmus, jerk see-saw nystagmus, oculogyric crisis, and ophthalmoplegia.

Gaze-Evoked Nystagmus

As commonly seen with other antiepileptic use, the gaze evoked nystagmus is also seen in patients who take carbamazepine. The mechanism of gaze-evoked nystagmus secondary to carbamazepine also involves the vestibulocerebellum or its connections [17, 18]. Further details regarding neuroanatomy and mechanism has ben discussed under the section of sodium valproate.

Slowed Saccades

Saccades are fast eye movements that redirect the point of fixation. Saccades matrix includes the eye fields in cerebral cortex, superior colliculus, and the brainstem saccadic pulse generator network. There are two types of neurons in the brainstem generator network: burst neurons and omnipause neurons. For horizontal saccades, the saccadic burst neurons are in the paramedian pontine reticular formation (PPRF) within the caudal pons. For vertical and torsional saccades, burst neurons are within the riMLF. There are two types of burst neurons, excitatory burst neurons and inhibitory burst neurons [19]. Activated excitatory burst neurons cause tonic firing of the associated extraocular muscle to perform a saccade. The inhibitory burst neurons' roles include silencing the activity in the antagonist extraocular muscles during saccades. Another role may be to help end the saccade when the eyes are on the target [20]. The duration of most saccades is less than 100 milliseconds and have a peak velocity of approximately 500 degrees/second. Carbamazepine may decrease peak saccade velocity. The mechanism is via the drug-induced dysfunction of the neuronal depolarization within the brainstem saccade pulse generator system in the PPRF [20].

Smooth Pursuit

Smooth pursuit movements are slower tracking movements of the eyes to keep a moving target on the fovea. Neuroanatomical structures involved for smooth pursuit include cerebral cortical areas, the neural integrator, and vestibulocerebellum. Further details are discussed previously.

The mechanism in which carbamazepine impairs smooth pursuit can be presumed similar to phenytoin as they have similar inhibitory actions on the sodium channels. The carbamazepine putatively inhibits vestibulocerebellum impairing smooth pursuit [21].

Downbeat Nystagmus

Downbeat nystagmus results from a defective vertical gaze holding causing a pathologic updrift of eyes and a corrective downward saccade. Downbeat nystagmus can be present in dysfunctions of the vestibulocerebellum as well. The induction of downbeat nystagmus by carbamazepine may reflect disruption of the cerebellum and its control of vestibular, pursuit, or otolith-ocular reflexes [22].

Seesaw Nystagmus

Seesaw nystagmus is relatively uncommon forms of nystagmus where one eye elevates and intorts while the other moves downwards and extorts. Factors that contribute to jerk seesaw nystagmus include imbalance and miscalibration of vestibular responses that normally optimize gaze during head rotations in roll. The vestibular nuclei will provide inputs to oculomotor and trochlear nuclei via the medial longitudinal fasciculus (MLF) to maintain gaze. Discoordination and miscalibration between these structures may manifest as seesaw nystagmus. Oxcarbazepine may disrupt the coordination of vestibular inputs to cause seesaw nystagmus [23].

Oculogyric Crisis

Oculogyric crisis is characterized by prolonged involuntary upward gaze deviation. Patients have great difficulty in looking downward as the eyes become fixed in an upward gaze. It is often associated as an acute dystonic reaction due to neuroleptic drug treatment. But it can sometimes be seen in carbamazepine use. This may be secondary to imbalance of the neural integrator and its vertical gaze-holding mechanism [24].

Ophthalmoplegia

One study described ophthalmoplegia induced by carbamazepine [25]. It is possible that global weakening of burst generation or profound and sustained inhibition by the omnipause neurons have caused the deficit. The omnipause neurons are located within the nucleus raphe interpositus which is located within the dorsal caudal pons. They exert a tonic inhibition upon horizontal and vertical saccadic burst neurons during fixation or smooth pursuit eye movements. Before a saccade is generated, the high level of tonic inhibition by the omnipause neurons is removed. The release of inhibition by omnipause neurons disinhibits the saccadic burst neurons which are then able to perform a saccade [26]. It is postulated that carbamazepine impairs the normal release of inhibition by omnipause neurons which leads to constant tonic inhibition of excitatory burst neuron manifesting as ophthalmoplegia.

Lamotrigine

The mechanism of action of lamotrigine is not fully elucidated as it may have multiple actions that likely contribute to its broad clinical efficacy. In regard to its anti-epileptic effect, lamotrigine is a member of the sodium channel blockade agents. Lamotrigine blocks voltage-activated sodium channels which decreases presynaptic release of excitatory neurotransmitters such as glutamate.

Downbeat Nystagmus

Lamotrigine toxicity can cause downbeat nystagmus. The presence of downbeat nystagmus supports the involvement of the vestibulocerebellum [27, 28].

Benzodiazepines and Barbiturates

Lorazepam, diazepam, clonazepam, clobazam, and others belong to the benzodiazepine family. They enhance the efficacy of the inhibitory neurotransmitter GABA at the $GABA_A$ receptor to decrease the neuronal excitability. The benzodiazepines act as a positive allosteric modulator and hyperpolarizes the neuronal membrane potential by increasing the chloride ion conductance. Barbiturates, such as phenobarbital and primidone, have a similar mechanism of action as benzodiazepines, they too potentiate the effects of GABA. Like benzodiazepines, barbiturates bind as a positive allosteric modulator to the $GABA_A$ receptor. At higher doses they act as $GABA_A$ agonists. Benzodiazepines increase the frequency of chloride channel opening whereas barbiturates increase the opening duration. In addition, barbiturates block the excitatory glutaminergic AMPA and kainate receptors. Taken together, barbiturates potentiate inhibitory $GABA_A$ receptors and inhibit excitatory AMPA receptors. Similar eye movement abnormalities arise in patients taking benzodiazepines or barbiturates. This may be due to their GABAergic properties. They include increase duration and decreased velocity of saccades and impaired smooth pursuit.

Saccade Duration and Velocity

During a saccade, a high-frequency burst of activity occurs in ocular motoneurons and its agonist ocular muscle. This burst of activity is the *saccadic pulse of innervation* and generates the force necessary to overcome the orbital viscous drag for the eyes to move. After the pulse of innervation to perform the saccade, the eyes are held in the new position by the orbital muscles countering the orbital elastic restoring forces. To hold the eyes in this new position after a saccade, a higher level of tonic innervation of the ocular motoneurons and its agonist orbital muscles is required and is termed the *saccadic step of innervation.* Meanwhile, reciprocal inhibitory changes occur in the antagonist orbital muscles and motoneurons to perform the saccade.

The neuroanatomy for saccade initiation includes the PPRF for horizontal saccades and riMLF for vertical and torsional saccades. Omnipause neurons (OPNs) within the nucleus raphe interpositus exert continuous inhibition upon all burst neurons for saccade generation in any direction. During saccade initiation, the high tonic inhibition of OPNs are released. This disinhibition of the burst neurons allows activation of ocular muscles resulting in a saccade. Moreover, superior colliculus regulates the OPNs and thus it has strong control over saccade generation.

Saccades necessitate a fine balance between inhibitory and excitatory activity as well as close interplay between structures throughout the brainstem, cerebellum, and cortical eye fields. Barbiturates and benzodiazepines can impair the neural network that generates saccades. This can result in reduced velocity, increased latency, and increased duration of saccades. The velocity of saccades are strongly related to the discharge rate of burst neurons in the PPRF. The firing rate of burst neurons might be affected by a person's level of consciousness as slower saccades occur in drowsiness. Benzodiazepines and barbiturates have sedating effects which alters the tonic firing of saccadic OPNs [29].

Additionally, there can also be increased saccade latencies. Diazepam increases the latencies of saccades in saccadic reaction time testing. This finding is attributed to the vigilance-lowering properties of diazepam and its effects on attention [30–32]. Another study found that serum concentrations of benzodiazepines, such as diazepam, also resulted in decreased peak horizontal saccadic velocity. This demonstrated a relationship between serum benzodiazepine concentration and its slowing and sedating effect on brainstem reticular formation function by measuring peak saccade velocity [33].

In conjunction with their sedative effects, the $GABA_A$ agonist activity of benzodiazepines and barbiturates may also influence the neural networks of saccades through the OPNs. The OPNs have GABAergic, glycinergic, and glutaminergic afferents. The inhibitory $GABA_A$ agonist activity of benzodiazepines may impair normal OPNs activity upon burst neurons and play a role in increased saccade latency and reduced peak saccade velocity [34].

Smooth Pursuit

Smooth pursuit neural matrix consists of cortex, pons, and cerebellum which then project to ocular motoneurons. Within the cerebellum, the dorsal vermis and paraflocculus receive inputs from the pons (dorsolateral pontine nucleus and nucleus reticularis tegmenti pontis) and the inferior olive. Then the dorsal vermis and paraflocculus project to the fastigial nucleus and vestibular nucleus which then provide outputs to the ocular motoneurons to perform smooth-pursuit eye movements.

The dorsal vermis and caudal fastigial nucleus contribute most to the onset of smooth pursuit while the vestibulocerebellum contributes most to steady-state tracking. Purkinje cells in the paraflocculus and flocculus modulate their discharge according to gaze velocity and eye position during smooth pursuit. The caudal fastigial nucleus receives inputs from the Purkinje cells of the dorsal vermis and axon collaterals from the pontine nuclei and discharge to initiate onset of smooth pursuit.

Impairment of smooth pursuit by benzodiazepines and barbiturates may be due to its effects on the cerebellum. The inhibitory GABAergic effects on the cerebellum may be the mechanism in which benzodiazepines and barbiturates impair smooth pursuit. Particularly, diazepam can reduce the amplitude (gain) of smooth pursuit eye tracking as well as decrease smooth pursuit velocity [35, 36].

Propofol and Midazolam

Propofol and midazolam are intravenous anesthetics commonly employed in the management of patients with status epilepticus. Both propofol and midazolam act upon $GABA_A$ receptors. Propofol increases GABA mediated inhibitory tone in the central nervous system by decreasing the rate of dissociation of GABA from the $GABA_A$ receptor. This results in hyperpolarization of cell membranes by increasing the opening duration of GABA-mediated chloride channels. At higher concentrations, propofol behaves as a $GABA_A$ receptor agonist by directly activating $GABA_A$ receptors in the absence of GABA. Midazolam also enhances the effect of GABA on the $GABA_A$ receptor by increasing the frequency of chloride channel opening resulting in neuronal hyperpolarization. Midazolam does not activate $GABA_A$ receptors directly, differing from the propofol at higher concentrations.

Saccade Latency and Velocity

The described eye movement abnormalities associated with both propofol and midazolam include increased latency and decreased peak velocity of saccades. Propofol has also been found to reduce ocular microtremor which is a small high frequency random tremor of the eyes linked to neural activity in the brainstem and reticular formation. The sedative effect can be attributed to their suppression of the brainstem reticular formation, which is supported by alterations in the ocular microtremor observed in anesthetized patients. Such sedative effect might also alter the tonic firing of the saccadic OPNs by altering the tone of their GABAergic afferents [37, 38].

Ictal Eye Movement Disorders

Eye and head movement abnormalities are common clinical manifestations of epileptic seizures.

Versive Seizures

Versive movements are characterized as sustained involuntary head and eye deviations. The eye movements typically precede the head movements in which the eyes first deviate laterally followed by head turning. Also, the deviation of the eyes can appear to move horizontally either in a stepwise fashion, or in a smooth and continuous manner. The direction of gaze deviation and head turning in a versive seizure can aid localization of the seizure focus. The direction of version typically occurs contralateral to the seizure focus but can also be ipsilateral. Version can also be seen in frontal, temporal, or occipital lobe foci. One distinguishing factor to aid localization of the seizure focus is if awareness is preserved during version. If awareness is maintained during versive seizures, the focus originates in the contralateral frontal lobe. Loss of awareness during versive seizures are more likely to occur with temporal lobe foci. In addition to loss of awareness in temporal lobe foci, the direction of version can either be ipsilateral or contralateral to the temporal lobe focus. This is in contrast to frontal lobe seizure foci which are typically contralateral to the direction of version. Frontal eye field activation causes the contralateral horizontal gaze deviation. The frontal eye field is located in the middle frontal gyrus and adjacent precentral gyrus, between Brodmann areas 4, 6 and 8. During the initiation of eye movements, such as voluntary saccades and pursuit movements, the frontal eye field is activated and provides information to the contralateral paramedian pontine reticular formation (PPRF) via the frontopontine fibers. From there, the medial longitudinal fasciculus (MLF) system is activated which coordinates horizontal eye movements by stimulating the oculomotor nucleus and its innervation to the medial rectus and the abducens nucleus and its innervation to the lateral rectus. In summary, the seizure can stimulate the ipsilateral frontal eye field which can cause contralateral horizontal gaze deviation via descending frontopontine fibers to activate the PPRF-MLF network. In this example, awareness is preserved. In contrast, versive seizures seen in temporal lobe epilepsy first has loss of awareness and later can stimulate the frontal eye field when the seizure spreads to the frontal lobe. In addition, version can be contralateral or ipsilateral to the temporal lobe seizure foci. The ipsilateral version may be due to seizure spread to the contralateral medial temporal lobe and further spread to cortical and subcortical structures of the frontal and parietal lobes. This spread may then stimulate the frontal eye field contralateral to the temporal lobe seizure focus and generate an ipsilateral versive seizure.

A similar mechanism of version is also seen in parietal and occipital lobe seizures. In these cases, the direction of version is typically contralateral, similar to frontal lobe seizures. It is also likely due to parietal eye field activation secondary to the seizure spread [39].

It was mentioned earlier that the versive eye movements can either be stepwise or smooth and continuous. This difference is dependent on the area within the frontal eye field that is activated. Stimulation studies performed on the frontal eye field results in different patterns of eye version. (Fig. 4.2) When the posterior portion of the frontal eye field is stimulated near the precentral gyrus, a contralateral smooth pursuit eye movement is seen. When the frontal eye field is stimulated more anteriorly, contralateral step-wise saccades are seen [40]. In addition to the step-wise or smooth pursuit eye movements seen with stimulation of different portions of the frontal eye field, there can also be a difference in the size of saccades as well. Stimulation of the ventrolateral portion of the frontal eye field generates shorter saccades whereas stimulation of the mediodorsal frontal eye field generates larger saccades [41].

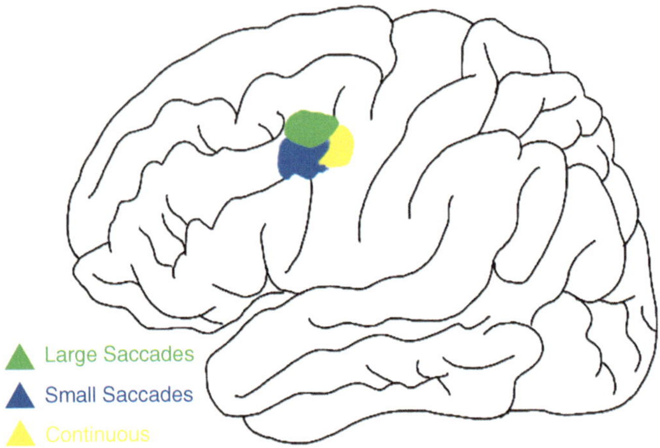

Fig. 4.2 Frontal Eye Field: Located at the caudal end of the middle frontal gyrus and anterior to the precentral gyrus. Posterior frontal eye field (blue) activation results in a contralateral smooth pursuit eye movement. Activation of the anterior frontal eye field results in contralateral step-wise saccades. If the anterior ventrolateral region of the frontal eye field (orange) is activated, shorter saccades are seen. If the anterior mediodorsal region of the frontal eye field (red) is activated, larger saccades are seen. (Reproduced with permission from Shaikh and Ghasia [52])

Epileptic Nystagmus

Epileptic nystagmus is due to epileptic activity which causes rapid, repetitive eye movements. If observed, it is a reliable sign localizing the epileptogenic zone to the contralateral hemisphere to the fast phase of nystagmus. The duration of epileptic nystagmus is usually short and persist less than 1 minute [42]. There are two proposed mechanisms for epileptic nystagmus. One involves epileptic activation of a cortical saccade region (frontal eye field, supplementary eye field, parietal eye field) causing contraversive quick phases combined with a defect in the gaze-holding system such as a leaky neural integrator. This allows the eyes to drift back toward the midline. In this situation, an epileptic discharge would cause a contraversive quick-phase eye movement followed by a slow phase caused by the leaky neural integrator (which is based upon an assumption of impaired neural integrator function secondary to AED use and is discussed further in the next paragraph) that would bring the eyes toward the midline of the orbit. Another mechanism involves epileptic activation of a cortical pursuit region (primary visual areas, temporo-parietal-occipital junction) generating an ipsiversive slow phase followed by a reflexive saccade as the eye reaches the far eccentric position in the orbit [43].

The proposed neural mechanism for epileptic nystagmus is based on the assumption of a leaky neural integrator. Many anti-epileptic medications such as phenytoin, phenobarbital, carbamazepine, and benzodiazepines can cause a leaky neural integrator. In patients found to have epileptic nystagmus, many had seizure activity within the temporo-parieto-occipital cortex and had high frequency epileptic discharges greater than 10 Hz. Epileptic nystagmus is rarely seen as these prerequisites are uncommonly met [43, 44].

Epileptic Monocular Nystagmus

Epileptic monocular nystagmus is an extremely rare phenomenon with an unclear mechanism. One report found epileptic monocular nystagmus provoked by intermittent photic stimulation in a cognitively impaired 15-year-old girl with poor visual acuity of the involved eye and generalized epilepsy. The authors concluded it was a pathologic form of flash-induced after-nystagmus [45]. Another report described epileptic monocular nystagmus in a patient with a right occipital lobe lesion secondary to Sturge-Weber syndrome. This patient had focal occipital lobe seizures contralateral to the involved eye. That patient's seizure semiology was limited to altered visual perceptions of the left hemifield and left eye, and left-beating epileptic monocular nystagmus. The authors provided a few proposed mechanisms. One was that the seizure discharge activated a cortical saccade region and caused simultaneous supranuclear inhibition of ipsilateral eye movement. Another proposed mechanism was based on the theory of von Helmholtz in that premotor eye movement commands are monocular and that the focal seizure discharge creates a monocular eye movement command at the cortical or brainstem level thus manifesting as epileptic monocular nystagmus [46]. Another study described ictal monocular nystagmus of the left eye secondary to a right frontal focal cortical dysplasia type 2b. In addition, there was also interictal monocular nystagmus of the right eye. The proposed hypothesis included not only focal cortical activation but also an irregular brainstem imbalance that overrides the regular binocular cortical and subcortical eye movement control mechanisms. The finding of interictal right eye monocular nystagmus may be due to a dysfunction of the right brainstem with possibly a "Todd's paralysis" of the analogous left brainstem nuclei due to high seizure frequency. In summary, this proposed hypothesis states that the simultaneous control of eye movements was transiently overridden by epileptic activity of the right frontal cortical focus exciting the right frontal eye field, stimulating cranial nerve nuclei III and VI in the ictal state, resulting in monocular nystagmus of the left eye. Then during the interictal state there was a monocular nystagmus of the right eye due to a presumed Todd's paralysis-like phenomenon of the left brainstem [47].

Ictal Eye Blinking

Ictal eye blinking is thought to occur from ictal cortical activity with descending activation of brainstem trigeminal fibers resulting in eye blinks [48]. Ictal unilateral blinking is considered a lateralizing sign to the ipsilateral hemisphere, typically being frontal but has been described secondary to ictal activity in other brain regions as well [49]. The pathway and mechanism for unilateral eye blinking are not well understood. Ipsilateral precentral, postcentral, temporal, and cerebellar regions as well as trigeminal fibers are thought to play a role in ipsilateral eye blinking. One proposed hypothesis is that ictal activity may pathologically inhibit the contralateral eye from blinking with descending inputs to trigeminal fibers causes blinking of the ipsilateral, non-inhibited eye [50]. Another proposed theory regarding ipsilateral eye blinking is based on stimulation studies of the dura. This hypothesis is based upon ictal activity stimulating trigeminal fibers coursing through and innervating subdural structures and pial vessels of the ipsilateral hemisphere which then unilaterally stimulates blinking of the ipsilateral eye [51].

Summary

In this chapter, we reviewed the abnormal eye movements in seizures and those caused by commonly used antiepileptics (AEDs). The goal of AEDs is to stabilize neuronal network and decreased the overall excitability in seizures. Hence abnormal eye movements can be observed in different AEDs due to their mechanism of action. (Table 4.1) Sodium valproate can cause gaze-evoke nys-

Table 4.1 Reproduced with permission from Shaikh and Ghasia [52]

AED	Mechanism of action	Eye movement abnormality	Mechanism of abnormality
Valproate	Na Channel Blocker	Gaze Evoked Nystagmus	Neural Integrator
	Increases GABA	Vertical Gaze Palsy	Deactivation of vertical burst neurons
Phenytoin	Na Channel Blocker	Gaze Evoked Nystagmus	Neural Integrator
		Impaired Smooth Pursuit	Vestibulocerebellum-Flocculus and Paraflocculus
		VOR Suppression	Vestibulocerebellum-Flocculus and Paraflocculus
		Downbeat Nystagmus	Vestibulocerebellum-Flocculus
		Periodic Alternating Nystagmus (PAN)	Vestibulocerebellum-Nodulus and Uvula
		Pendular Nystagmus	Neural Integrator

(continued)

Table 4.1 (continued)

AED	Mechanism of action	Eye movement abnormality	Mechanism of abnormality
Carbamazepine	Na Channel Blocker	Gaze Evoked Nystagmus	Neural Integrator
		Slowed Saccades	PPRF (burst neurons)
		Impaired Smooth Pursuit	Vestibulocerebellum
		Downbeat Nystagmus	Vestibulocerebellum-Flocculus
		Seesaw Nystagmus	Vestibular inputs and gaze holding
		Oculogyric Crisis	Neural Integrator and vertical gaze holding
		Ophthalmoplegia	Omnipause Neurons
Lamotrigine	Na Channel Blocker	Downbeat Nystagmus	Vestibulocerebellum-Flocculus
Benzodiazepines	Enhances GABA	Slowed Saccades	PPRF (burst neurons) and OPNs
Barbiturates	Enhances GABA, AMPA Antagnoist	Impaired Smooth Pursuit	Vestibulocerebellum-Vermis and Flocculus
Propofol midazolam	Enhances GABA	Slowed Saccades	PPRF and OPNs

tagmus (GEN) and vertical gaze palsy. Whereas phenytoin/fosphenytoin can lead to GEN, downbeat nystagmus, periodic alternating nystagmus (PAN) and pendular nystagmus. They also affect smooth pursuit and vestibulo-ocular reflex function. Carbamazepine can cause similar abnormalities like phenytoin. Additionally, seesaw nystagmus, oculogyric crisis and ophthalmoplegia were also reported to be induced by it. Lamotrigine is known to cause downbeat nystagmus. Benzodiazepines and barbiturates might increase saccade latency and lower its velocity. Seizures can manifest as abnormal eye movements at times. Most observed eye movement abnormality is gaze deviation, which is a valuable localizing sign for the seizure focus. Epileptic nystagmus is a rare manifestation, if observed, also provides important localization value for the seizure focus. In rare occasions, the nystagmus might happen only in one eye – epileptic monocular nystagmus. Ictal blinking was also reported in some seizure patients, which usually happens ipsilateral to the epileptic focus.

References

1. Sanchez K, Rowe FJ. Role of neural integrators in oculomotor systems: a systematic narrative literature review. Acta Ophthalmol. 2016;96(2):e111–8.
2. Suzuki Y, Kase M, Hashimoto M, et al. Leaky neural integration observed in square-wave jerks. Jpn J Ophthalmol. 2003;47:535–6.
3. Glassauer S, Hoshi M, Kempermann U, et al. Three-dimensional eye position and slow phase velocity in humans with downbeat nystagmus. J Neurophysiol. 2003;89:338–54.
4. Rett D. Gaze-evoked nystagmus: a case report and literature review. Optometry. 2007;78:460–4.
5. Zaccara G, Cincotta M, Borgheresi A, Balestrieri F. Adverse motor effects induced by antiepileptic drugs. Epileptic Disord. 2004;6(3):153–68.
6. Zee DS, Yee RD, Cogan DG, Robinson DA, Engel WK. Ocular motor abnormalities in hereditary cerebellar ataxia. Brain. 1976;99(2):207–34.
7. Horn AKE, Helmchen C, Wahle P. GABAergic neurons in the rostral mesencephalon of the macaque monkey that control vertical eye movements. Ann N Y Acad Sci. 2003;1004:19–28.
8. Gosala Raja KS, Srinivas M, Raghunandan N, et al. Reversible vertical gaze palsy in sodium valproate toxicity. J Neuroophthalmol. 2013;33:202–3.
9. Riker WK, Downes H, Olsen GD, et al. Conjugate lateral gaze nystagmus and free phenytoin concentrations in plasma: lack of correlation. Epilepsia. 1978;19:93–8.
10. Belton T, McCrea RA. Role of the cerebellar flocculus region in cancellation of the VOR during passive whole body rotation. J Neurophysiol. 2000;84:1599–613.
11. Bittencourt PR, Gresty MA, Richens A. Quantitative assessment of smooth-pursuit eye movements in healthy and epileptic subjects. J Neurol Neurosurg Psychiatry. 1980;43:1119–24.
12. Berger JR, Kovacs AG. Downbeat nystagmus with phenytoin. J Clin Neuroophthalmol. 1982;2:209–11.
13. Cohen B, Helwig D, Raphan T. Baclofen and velocity storage: a model of the effects of the drug on the vestibulo-ocular reflex in the rhesus monkey. J Physiol. 1987;393:703–25.

14. Campbell WW. Periodic alternating nystagmus in phenytoin intoxication. Arch Neurol. 1980;37:178–80.
15. Schwankhaus JD, Kattah JC, Lux WE, et al. Primidone/phenobarbital-induced periodic alternating nystagmus. Ann Ophthalmol. 1989;21:230–2.
16. Shaikh AG. Fosphenytoin induced transient pendular nystagmus. J Neurol Sci. 2013;330:121–2.
17. Umeda Y, Sakata E. Equilibrium disorder in carbamazepine toxicity. Ann Otol Rhinol Laryngol. 1977;86:318–22.
18. Remler BF, Leigh RJ, Osorio I, et al. The characteristics and mechanisms of visual disturbance associated with anticonvulsant therapy. Neurology. 1990;40:791–6.
19. Büttner Ennever JA, Büttner U. The reticular formation. In: Büttner-Enever JA, editor. Neuroanatomy of the oculomotor system. New York: Elsevier; 1988. p. 119–76.
20. Tedeschi G, Casucci G, Allocca S, et al. Neuroocular side effects of carbamazepine and phenobarbital in epileptic patients as measured by saccadic eye movements analysis. Epilepsia. 1989;30:62–6.
21. Reilly JL, Lencer R, Bishop JR, Keedy S, Sweeney JA. Pharmacological treatment effects on eye movement control. Brain Cogn. 2008;68(3):415–35. https://doi.org/10.1016/j.bandc.2008.08.026.
22. Chrousos GA, Cowdry R, Schuelein M, et al. Two cases of downbeat nystagmus and oscillopsia associated with carbamazepine. Am J Ophthalmol. 1987;103:221–4.
23. Adamec I, Nankovic S, Zadro I, et al. Oxcarbazepine-induced jerky see-saw nystagmus. Neurol Sci. 2013;34:1839–40.
24. Berchou RC, Rodin EA. Carbamazepine-induced oculogyric crisis. Arch Neurol. 1979;36:522–3.
25. Noda S, Umezaki H. Carbamazepine-induced ophthalmoplegia. Neurology. 1982;32:1320.
26. Horn AK, Büttner-Ennever JA, Wahle P, Reichenberger I. Neurotransmitter profile of saccadic omnipause neurons in nucleus raphe interpositus. J Neurosci. 1994;14:2032–46.
27. Oh SY, Kim JS, Lee YH, et al. Downbeat, positional, and perverted head-shaking nystagmus associated with lamotrigine toxicity. J Clin Neurol. 2006;2:283–5.
28. Alkawi A, Kattah JC, Wyman K. Downbeat nystagmus as a result of lamotrigine toxicity. Epilepsy Res. 2005;63:85–8.
29. Keller EL. Control of saccadic eye movements by midline brain stem neurons. In: Baker R, Berthoz A, editors. Control of gaze by brain stem neurons. Amsterdam: Elsevier; 1977. p. 327–36.
30. Fafrowicz M, Unrug A, Marek T, et al. Effects of diazepam and buspirone on reaction time of saccadic eye movements. Neuropsychobiology. 1995;32:156–60.
31. Rothennberg SJ, Selkoe D. Specific oculomotor deficit after diazepam. I. Saccadic eye movements. Psychopharmacology. 1981;74:232–6.

32. Masson GS, Mestre DR, Martineau F, et al. Lorazepam-induced modifications of saccadic and smooth-pursuit eye movements in humans: attentional and motor factors. Behav Brain Res. 2000;108:169–80.
33. Bittencourt PR, Wade P, Smith AT, et al. The relationship between peak velocity of saccadic eye movements and serum benzodiazepine concentration. Br J Clin Pharmacol. 1981;12:523–33.
34. Jürgens R, Becker W, Kornhuber HH. Natural and drug-induced variations of velocity and duration of human saccadic eye movements: evidence for a control of the neural pulse generator by local feedback. Biol Cybern. 1981;39:87–96.
35. Rothenberg SJ, Selkoe D. Specific oculomotor deficit after diazepam. II. Smooth pursuit eye movements. Psychopharmacology. 1981;74:237–40.
36. Bittencourt PR, Wade P, Smith AT, et al. Benzodiazepines impair smooth pursuit eye movements. Br J Clin Pharmacol. 1983;15:259–62.
37. Busettini C, Frolich MA. Effects of mild to moderate sedation on saccadic eye movements. Behav Brain Res. 2014;272:286–302.
38. Bojanic S, Simpson T, Bolger C. Ocular microtremor: a tool for measuring depth of anaesthesia? Br J Anaesth. 2001;86:519–22.
39. McLachlan RS. The significance of head and eye turning in seizures. Neurology. 1987;37(10):1617–9.
40. Schall JD. Frontal eye fields. In: Encyclopedia of neuroscience. Amsterdam: Elsevier BV; 2009. p. 367–74.
41. Milea D, Lobel E, Lehéricy S, et al. Intraoperative frontal eye field stimulation elicits ocular deviation and saccade suppression. Neuroreport. 2002;13(10):1359–64.
42. Ma Y, Wang J, Li D, Lang S. Two types of isolated epileptic nystagmus: case report. Int J Clin Exp Med. 2015;8(8):13500–7.
43. Kaplan PW, Tusa RJ. Neurophysiologic and clinical correlations of epileptic nystagmus. Neurology. 1993;43:2508–14.
44. Kellinghaus C, Skidmore C, Loddenkemper T. Lateralizing value of epileptic nystagmus. Epilepsy Behav. 2008;13:700–2.
45. Jacome DE, FitzGerald R. Monocular ictal nystagmus. Arch Neurol. 1982;39:653–6.
46. Grant AC, Jain V, Bose S. Epileptic monocular nystagmus. Neurology. 2002;59:1438–41.
47. Schulz R, Tomka-Hoffmeister M, Woermann FG, et al. Epileptic monocular nystagmus and ictal diplopia as cortical and subcortical dysfunction. Epilepsy Behav Case Rep. 2013;1:89–91.
48. Saporito MAN, Vitaliti G, Pavone P, et al. Ictal blinking, an underrecognized phenomenon: our experience and literature review. Neuropsychiatr Dis Treat. 2017;13:1435–9.
49. Kalss G, Leitinger M, Dobesberger J, Granbichler CA, Kuchukhidze G, Trinka E. Ictal unilateral eye blinking and contralateral blink inhibition - a video-EEG study and review of the literature. Epilepsy Behav Case Rep. 2013;1:161–5.

50. Kalss G, Leitinger M, Dobesberger J, Granbichler CA, Kuchukhidze G, Trinka E. Ictal unilateral eye blinking and contralateral blink inhibition - a video-EEG study and review of the literature. Epilepsy Behav Case Rep. 2013;1:161–5.
51. Falsaperla R, Perciavalle V, Pavone P, et al. Unilateral eye blinking arising from the ictal ipsilateral occipital area. Clin EEG Neurosci. 2014;47(3):243–6.
52. Shaikh AG, Ghasia FF, editors. Advances in translational neuroscience of eye movement disorders. Cham: Springer; 2019.

Eye Movements in Coma

5

The eye movement examination of unconscious patients may aid diagnosis and prognosis [1]. The mainstay of ocular motor examination in the comatose patients include observation of eyelid movements, spontaneous eye movements during resting, and reflexive eye movements.

Eyelid Movements

The eyelids are typically closed in coma, but unlike sleep or voluntary eye closure, there is no tonic contraction of the eyelids. Lift and release of the eyelid during passive eye opening is free of resistance [2]. Spontaneous movements of the eyelids can be seen in patients with spontaneous vertical eye movements. Due to yoked nature of superior rectus with levator palpabre superiororis, the downbeat nystagmus is associated with downward jerky movement of the eyelid; the opposite is seen with upbeat nystagmus. The lid movements can be present in those with ongoing seizure or be part of epilepsia partialis continua. Two types of lid movements, lid saccades and blinks, have discrete kinematic properties and physiology. These differences are reflected in distinct phenomenology of the disorders affecting their neural substrate. The lid movements in the patient with parietal lobe epilepsy can be rhythmic, yoked, and have a fast-upward component that

A. Shaikh, F. Wang, *Eye Movements in the Critical Care Setting*,
https://doi.org/10.1007/978-3-030-70221-2_5

instantaneously follow a slow downward passive drift. These cyclic movements strikingly resemble nystagmus, but unlike nystagmus, the fast-upward component is pathological and supported by the saccadic mechanism. Furthermore, ipsilateral rapid downward lid movement resembling reflex or blink can also be seen in those with active ongoing seizures.

Spontaneous Eye Movements

The spontaneous eye movements in the comatose patients can be broadly classified into two types; those exclusively present in comatose patients and the ones that are non-exclusive but either pre-existing or exacerbated due to the underlying pathology leading to coma.

Spontaneous Eye Movements That Are Exclusive to Comatose State

Conjugate gaze deviation or ocular misalignment provide useful information in comatose patients (Table 5.1).

Horizontal conjugate eye deviation is frequently seen in unconscious patients, the location of the eyes sometimes provides the diagnostic clue to the underlying pathology. When a hemispheric deficit is above the level of the basal ganglia, the eyes deviate to the lesion side. The mechanistic underpinning for such deviation direction is imbalanced inputs from two frontal eye fields. The cortical deficits leading to conjugate eye deviation reverses in those whose brain is stimulated. For example, seizures cause overactivation of one cortical eye field and make the eyes deviate to the contralateral side. In latter scenario it is possible to have nystagmus with fast phase directed contralesionally. However, at the end of cortical seizure, the eyes drift towards the ipsilesional side, i.e., the Todd's paralysis of the extraocular muscles [3, 4]. Very rarely, supratentorial hemorrhage or extensive hemispheric infarct cause eyes deviation away from the lesion [5–8]. Such deficits

Table 5.1 Spontaneous Eye Movements in Unconsciousness

Horizontal Deviation	**Ipsilesional:** Hemispheric injury (infarct, hemorrhage, Todd's paralysis, etc.) Horizontal gaze-evoked nystagmus on looking contralaterally Wallenberg syndrome (lateropulsion) Vestibular nucleus injury (vascular, compression) **Contralesional:** Seizure Hemispheric ischemic or hemorrhagic lesion (rarely) Thalamic hemorrhage Pontine lesion (especially involving paramedian pontine tegmentum) Inferior olivary nucleus lesion
Downward Deviation	Thalamic hemorrhage Rostral dorsal midbrain injury Metabolic encephalopathy (including hypoxic ischemic encephalopathy, intoxication) Feigned coma seizures
Upward Deviation	Hypoxic ischemic encephalopathy Oculogyric crisis Eyes-open comma (rarely)

suggest cerebral edema or "subclinical" seizures secondary to the primary lesion. The thalamic hemorrhages or pontine tegmentum lesions can cause contralateral gaze deviation, i.e., the "wrong way eyes." [9, 10] Further down in the brainstem, inferior olive, fastigial nucleus and vestibular nucleus forms a complete circuit and lesion within the circuit could also lead to conjugate eye deviation, but the deviation could be in either direction contingent upon the location of primary injury. For example, the Wallenberg syndrome cause ipsilateral conjugate eye deviation due to the lesions affecting the inferior cerebellar peduncle [11, 12]. The lesions affecting inferior olive can cause contralateral conjugate eye deviation [13]. The involvement of cerebellar peduncles and tightly spaced brainstem nuclei can be seen in those with space occupying masses in the posterior fossa although the primary location of the mass may not be in the region concerned with eye movement control.

The vertical eye deviations are also not uncommon. The Fig. 5.1 depicts the neural substrate for the downward eye movement. Tonic downward deviation, associated with convergence appearing as "peering at the tip of the nose" is commonly seen in patients with thalamic hemorrhage [14, 15] Such deficits can also be seen in the Parinaud syndrome. Metabolic encephalopathy and hypoxic ischemic encephalopathy can also cause sustained downward gaze deviation [16, 17]. Sustained downgaze in hypoxic ischemic encephalopathy predicts poor prognosis and suggest diffuse cerebellar injury [18]. Seizures can also lead to tonic downgaze deviation [19].

Tonic upgaze deviation is commonly seen in hypoxic ischemic encephalopathy typically within hours after cardiac arrest [18, 20, 21]. Figure 5.2 demonstrated the neural substrates for upward eye movements. The upward deviation is due to the lack of inhibition from the cerebellum to the brainstem anterior semicircular canal

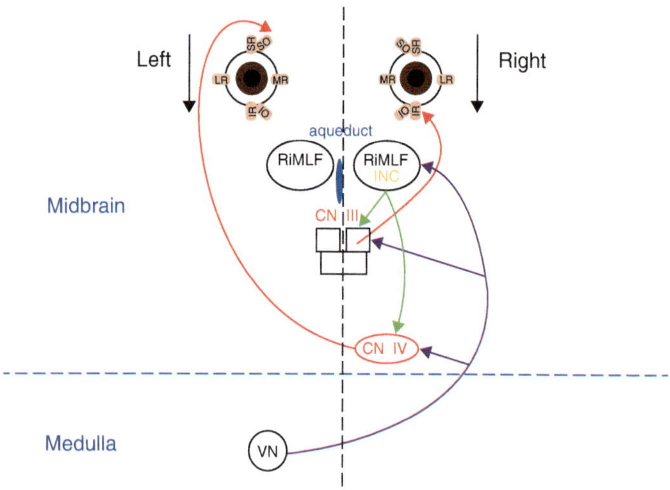

Fig. 5.1 Illustration of the neural substrate for downward eye movements. Vestibular nucleus (VN) sends signals to IIIrd and IVth nucleus, rostral insterstitial nucleus of medial longitudinal fasciculus (riMLF) and interstitial nucleus of Cajal (INC). riMLF and INC have ipsilateral projections to the IIIrd and IVth nucleus to adjust downward eye movements

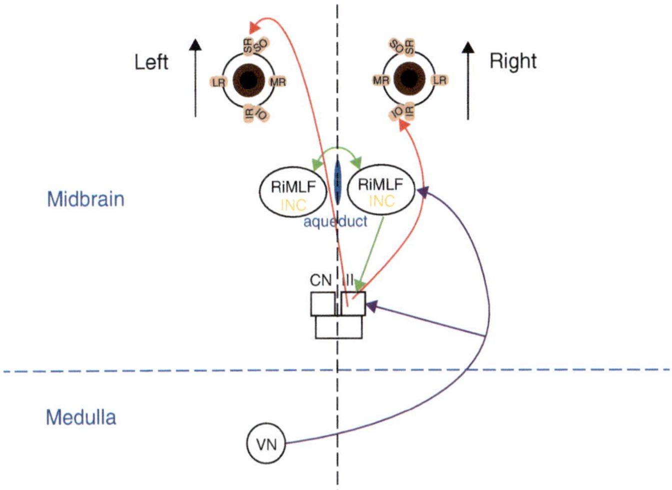

Fig. 5.2 Illustration of the neural substrate for upward eye movements. Vestibular nucleus (VN) sends projections to the IIIrd nucleus group, riMLF and INC. The bilateral riMLF and INC exchange signals via posterior commissure. They then project to the IIIrd nucleus to facilitate upward eye movements

projections secondary to diffuse cerebellar injury [22, 23]. The Fig. 5.3 proposed the pathophysiology of such change. Conversely, some patients may develop downward gaze deviation at later stage [18]. Oculogyric crises, another cause of upgaze deviation in critically ill patients, can be seen as a result of intoxication secondary to dopamine receptor blockade [24–34]. These unconscious patients can have spastic eyelids leading to sustained eye opening with upward deviated gaze [35]. It is postulated that pontomesencephalic damage causes disrupted eyelid relaxation; the upward gaze deviation possibly reflects preserved Bell's phenomenon.

It is not uncommon to find exophoria in unconscious patient. Other types of misalignments could also be observed in unconscious patients. For example, patients with internuclear ophthalmoplegia (INO) or oculomotor nerve palsy can have exotropia of the affected eye. The sixth nerve palsy can cause esotropia. The vertical misalignment is likely due to skew deviation, oculomotor or trochlear nerve palsy.

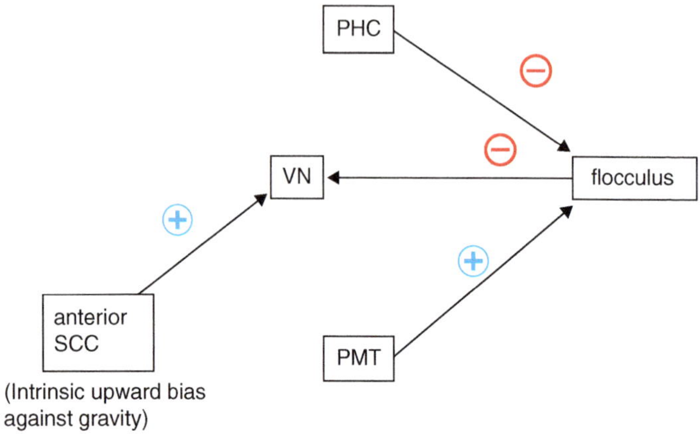

Fig. 5.3 The simplified version of the floccular pathway is illustrated. Anterior semicircular canal (anterior SCC) has intrinsic upward bias signal to make up for gravity pull. The flocculus is the integrator receiving signals from perihypoglossal complex (PHC) and the paramedian tract cell groups (PMT). The flocculus normally inhibits the vestibular nucleus (VN) to balance the intrinsic upward bias signal from anterior SCC

Spontaneous Eye Movements in Unconscious Patients

There are a wide variety of spontaneous eye movements that could be observed in unconscious patients, we summarized the common findings and causes in the following table (Table 5.2).

Ocular bobbing and its variants are some of the typical presentations of spontaneous eye movements in an unconscious patient.

Ocular bobbing is described as conjugate rapid downward movements followed by a slow return to the central gaze at an irregular rate [36–39] (Fig. 5.4). However, sometimes disconjugate eye movements are also seen [40]. Disconjugacy in ocular bobbing may suggest central pathology disrupting yoked nature of the eye movements. Ocular bobbing, historically considered a classic finding secondary to the pontine lesions, was later also described in the cerebellar lesions, metabolic and toxic encephalopathy, encephalitis, or hypoxic ischemic encephalopathy [41–47]. The neural mechanism still remains unclear, but

Table 5.2 Spontaneous Eye Movements in Unconsciousness

Typical Ocular Bobbing	Pontine lesion (characteristically) Cerebellar lesion Metabolic toxic encephalopathy Hypoxic ischemic encephalopathy (HIE)
Ocular Dipping (Inverse Bobbing)	HIE, metabolic toxic encephalopathy Status epilepticus (both convulsive and nonconvulsive) Creutzfeldt-Jakob disease (CJD)
Reverse Ocular Bobbing	Metabolic toxic encephalopathy Encephalitis
Reverse Ocular Dipping (Converse Bobbing)	Metabolic toxic encephalopathy
Oculopalatal Tremor	Any lesion that disrupts Guillain-Mollaret triangle (vascular, autoimmune disorder)
Roving Eye Movements (Ping-pong gaze)	Diffuse bi-hemispheric process (e.g. metabolic encephalopathy, HIE, post-ictal state)
Periodic Alternating Gaze Deviation (PAGD)	Cerebellar nodular lesions CJD Hepatic encephalopathy Posterior reversible encephalopathy syndrome (PRES)
Downbeat Nystagmus	Any lesion involving vestibulocerebellum or its input (vascular, autoimmune, neoplastic) Wernicke's encephalopathy
Upbeat Nystagmus	Any lesion involving brainstem, particularly caudal paramedian medulla Wernicke's encephalopathy
Torsional Nystagmus	Any lesion involving brainstem or cerebellum (vascular, autoimmune, neoplastic)
Seesaw and Hemi-seesaw Nystagmus	Pathology involving visual pathway Any lesion involving brainstem and cerebellum (vascular, autoimmune, neoplastic)

three hypotheses were proposed [48]. One hypothesis suggested ocular bobbing is an acute manifestation of inferior olive oscillation due to lack of inhibitory influence from the central tegmental tract injury in pontine lesions. The weakness of this hypothesis is that the oscillations from inferior olive typically have 2 Hz fundamental frequency, while ocular bobbing can have a frequency much slower than 2 Hz. Typically, oscillation of eyes in

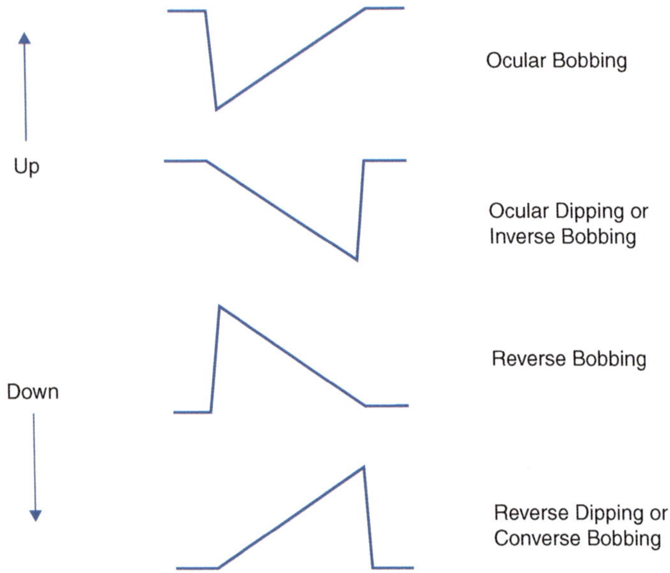

Fig. 5.4 Schematic representation of ocular bobbing and its variants. Ocular bobbing has rapid downward movements followed by a slow return to the central gaze. Ocular dipping is the inverse of ocular bobbing, hence inverse bobbing. Reverse bobbing starts with rapid upward movements followed by slow return to the central gaze. Reverse dipping is the mirror version of reverse bobbing; hence it starts with slow upward drifts followed by rapid return to the baseline

inferior olive hypertrophy is accompanied with palate oscillation, but palatal myoclonus is not typically present in comatose subjects with ocular bobbing. Lastly, the coarse ocular oscillation in the syndrome of inferior olive is attributed to initial pseudohypertrophy leading to hypersynchrony and secondly maladaptive conditional learning in the cerebellum to make the discharges coarse and disconjugate; all these phenomena take much longer time to develop. Moreover, it was also proposed that the convergent-divergent component of ocular bobbing, when present, may suggest involvement of the pretectal plate in the midbrain [49–51]. Furthermore, role of unstable neural integrator was also suggested. Paramedian tract cell groups (PMT), under normal circumstances, excite the cerebellar flocculus which is instrumental in providing feedback to brainstem neural integrators. The PMT lesions may cause unstable neural integrator with increased slow-phase velocity waveforms of the ocular bobbing [52]. Complete pathophysiology to support the neural integrator hypothesis remains to be further examined. Such focal deficit also does not explain ocular bobbing in those with diffuse metabolic encephalopathy or hypoxic ischemic encephalopathy. Lastly, it was also proposed that it results from the injury to the omnipause neurons, which then causes saccadic intrusions. However, the manifestations expected from the omnipause neuron injury are much more different in most cases. Additionally, they also demonstrate slow saccades and absence of nystagmus quick phase. Those deficits do not always manifest in the comatose patients with ocular bobbing.

Ocular dipping, or inverse bobbing, is characterized by an initial slow downward movement followed by a rapid jerk back to the central position (Fig. 5.4). Ocular dipping often spares horizontal reflexive eye movements or roving horizontal movements [53]. The ocular dipping has been reported in those with hypoxic ischemic encephalopathy, metabolic toxic encephalopathy, status epilepticus (both convulsive and nonconvulsive) and Creutzfeldt-Jakob disease (CJD) [47, 53, 55–63]. The synchrony between the eyelids and vertical eye movements can be preserved [54]. Tactile or noxious stimulation are typical provoking maneuvers of ocular dipping.

Reverse ocular bobbing is another variant of ocular bobbing described as rapid upward deviation of the eyes with a slow return to central position [64] (Fig. 5.4). This phenomenology usually indicates diffuse brain injury due to metabolic toxic encephalopathy or encephalitis [64–66]. Synchrony with eyelids is often one of the features of reverse ocular bobbing [66].

Reverse ocular dipping, or converse bobbing, is the last variant of ocular bobbing described as a slow upward drift of eyes followed by quick jerk back to central position [56, 64, 66–69] (Fig. 5.4). Similarly, there are only limited case reports to date, and its presence conveys limited localization or prognostication value. Reverse ocular dipping is reported in metabolic toxic encephalopathy, and similarly the upward movements could also synchronize with eyelid movements [66].

The roving eye movements are frequently observed in patients with coma. They are typically horizontal but can be omnidirectional sometimes. Pure horizontal roving eye movements, i.e., ping-pong gaze, are slow random deviations of the eyes in encephalopathic or sedated state [1, 70]. The oscillations of roving eye movements have a wide variation in frequency ranging up to 8 seconds to complete one cycle [71]. Although the pathophysiology of the roving eye movements remains unclear, they are commonly seen in metabolic encephalopathy and may suggest weakened cortical control of the gaze. The roving eye movements may disappear as the coma deepens, which supports the hypothesis of disconnection between both hemispheres and the integral brainstem [72–80].

Periodic alternating gaze deviation is another form of cyclic conjugate gaze deviation with a cycle duration from 2 to 5 minutes [81, 82]. It is thought to share the same physiological mechanism as periodic alternating nystagmus (PAN) but only possess the slow components of PAN. The lack of fast phase suggests disruption of saccade pathways in the brainstem [83–85]. Such hypothesis is supported by the etiologies localized in the cerebellum or supratentorial space, including Creutzfeldt-Jacob disease, hepatic encephalopathy, and posterior reversible encephalopathy syndrome [81, 82, 84–87].

Spontaneous Eye Movements that Are Non-exclusive of Comatose State

It is not unusual for patients admitted to intensive care units to have preexisting neurological conditions that are previously compensated. The neurological or metabolic insult results in decompensated state exacerbating the preexisting conditions. Various forms of spontaneous nystagmus can fall into this category. It is also possible that spontaneous nystagmus and coma share a common etiology, and both are new in onset.

Downbeat nystagmus suggests several disease processes involving the cerebellum and its connections. In the critical care unit, the downbeat nystagmus may suggest either a pre-existing lesion in the brainstem-cerebellar circuit worsened by critically ill state or an acute lesion affecting the aforementioned circuit. It is critical to separate downbeat nystagmus with ocular dipping, latter typically has much lower velocity during the slow phase and longer cycle duration. In contrast, downbeat nystagmus appears more robustly oscillatory and much faster in velocity. If the patient can participate in the neurological exam, it may be helpful to determine the gaze orientation dependence of the downbeat nystagmus. Often the amplitude of downbeat nystagmus amplifies in the lateral gaze, and its amplitude depend on the vertical orientation of the eye position. Shared lesion location of downbeat and gaze evoked nystagmus often results in their coexistence. The aggregated trajectories of the downbeat and gaze evoked nystagmus produce a diagonal eye movement. Downbeat nystagmus often calls for a need to obtain brain imaging, preferably the MRI to investigate potential pathology in posterior fossa. Although the most common cause of downbeat nystagmus is still unknown, i.e., idiopathic, frequently posterior fossa stroke or multiple sclerosis attack can all result in such deficit. Wernicke's encephalopathy can also cause downbeat nystagmus; hence it may be beneficial to treat these patients with thiamine repletion.

Like downbeat, the upbeat nystagmus may also suggest a preexisting etiology that is exacerbated or the consequence of the lesion that has caused critically ill state. The localization value of the upbeat nystagmus is relatively limited compared to downbeat nystagmus, but it can be mapped to the brainstem lesions involving the medulla, midbrain, or pons [88–100]. Upbeat nystagmus can obey Alexander's law, have largest amplitude in the downward gaze, but not always [101]. Role of neural integrator in the pathogenesis of upbeat nystagmus has been suggested. Stroke is the most frequent cause of upbeat nystagmus in the critical care unit. It is not uncommon for Wernicke's encephalopathy to present with upbeat nystagmus as well [102, 103]. It is essential to pursue neuro imaging studies when upbeat nystagmus is discovered.

Torsional nystagmus can be present in the critically ill patient who is suffering from the stroke or other structural lesions affecting the midbrain or the cerebellum. The pure torsional nystagmus was also reported from the lesion within the medulla or cerebellar peduncles [104, 105]. While examining an unconscious patient, it is necessary to request a brain imaging if torsional nystagmus is identified.

Seesaw and hemi-seesaw nystagmus are relatively uncommon forms of nystagmus where one eye elevates and intorts while the other moves downwards and extorts [106–113]. Seesaw nystagmus has been reported in association with a variety of central disorders, such as parasellar tumors. Parasellar mass can lead to visual field disturbance and midbrain compression [106, 114]. Either asymmetric compression of vertical and torsional saccade generators or even loss of vision alone was postulated to be the cause of seesaw nystagmus [115–117]. The seesaw nystagmus was also reported to be part of ocular tilt reaction secondary to disruption of the ascending vestibular projections from the labyrinth via contralateral medial longitudinal fasciculus to the contralateral interstitial nucleus of Cajal [108, 109, 118, 119].

Reflexive Eye Movements in Unconscious Patients

Reflexive eye movements and their abnormalities provide additional diagnostic and prognostic value about the brainstem function. The vestibulo-ocular reflex (VOR) and optokinetic reflexes (OKN) are two primary mechanisms utilizing the same final common pathway under cerebellar influence, though their afferent pathways are discrete. The VOR depends upon the integrity of the vestibular end-organs while OKN is visually driven. Both can be reliably performed in the comatose patients, and their abnormalities can suggest specific structural injuries.

The accurate evaluation of the VOR requires a rapid head impulse to one side while observing the motion of the eyeball. In comatose patients, it is possible to find central conjugate ocular drift after passive lateral head movements; this phenomenon suggests abnormal neural integration. Presence of vertical eye movements in addition to the horizontal VOR during horizontal head impulse maneuvers, or vice versa, suggests lack of directional modulation typically indicating cerebellar abnormalities. Hypoactive VOR certainly indicates the peripheral end-organ damage or the lesion involves in the vestibular nerve or nucleus. Cerebellar lesions can also lead to hyperactive VOR. The VOR may be sluggish in patients with deep coma, with grave brainstem lesions, or under deep sedation. In such cases, caloric test with ice water can be more effective, due to its sustained stimulation and the arousing effects of the cold water.

Presence of vertical or horizontal VOR accounts for the normal brainstem function. However, absent VOR may be explained by structural causes or metabolic toxic etiologies [120, 121]. Ophthalmoplegia is another reason for absence of the VOR. Bilateral complete ophthalmoplegia in an comatose patient should prompt consideration for Guillain-Barré syndrome (Miller-Fisher variant), neuromuscular junction disorders, or Wernicke's encephalopathy [122]. Midbrain injury or lesions involving bilateral medial longitudinal fasciculus can abolish vertical VOR, while impaired horizontal VOR with intact vertical components may be seen in those with pontine tegmental lesions [123]. Impaired adduction in response to VOR is possible in patients with metabolic toxic encephalopathy [124–129]. Barbiturate coma may present with downward gaze deviation in response to caloric testing or absence of VOR [130]. Convergence retraction nystagmus can be seen in response to caloric stimulation in the patient with pineal tumor [131]. The reflexive eye movements, together with other clinical signs, are helpful for the prognostication of comatose patients.

Summary

In this chapter, we reviewed abnormal eye movements in coma from three perspectives – eyelid movements, spontaneous eye movements and reflexive eye movements. In comatose patients, eyelids are generally closed, however sometimes spontaneous eyelid movements might be noticed synchronizing with underlying eye movements. Spontaneous eye movements that are exclusive to comatose state are horizontal deviation, downward deviation and upward deviation. Vertical gaze deviation can be caused by a variety of reasons including hypoxic ischemic encephalopathy, metabolic encephalopathy, etc. Horizontal gaze deviation is commonly observed in hemispheric injury and seizures. Other types of spontaneous eye movements observed in unconscious patients include ocular bobbing and its variants, roving eye movements, periodic alternating gaze deviation, upbeat nystagmus, downbeat nystagmus, torsional nystagmus, seesaw and hemi-seesaw nystagmus, and oculopalatal tremor. And these abnormal eye movements can be observed in patients with preserved consciousness. As far as the reflexive eye movements – optokinetic nystagmus and vestibulo-ocular reflex, their presence is a reassuring sign indicating the integrity of underlying brainstem structure.

References

1. Posner JB, Plum F, Saper CB, Schiff N. Plum and Posner's diagnosis of stupor and coma. Oxford, NY: OUP; 2007.
2. van Ommen HJ, Thibaut A, Vanhaudenhuyse A, Heine L, Charland-Verville V, Wannez S, et al. Resistance to eye opening in patients with disorders of consciousness. J Neurol. 2018;265(6):1376–80.
3. Thurston SE, Leigh RJ, Osorio I. Epileptic gaze deviation and nystagmus. Neurology. 1985;35(10):1518–21.
4. Luders H, Vaca GF, Akamatsu N, Amina S, Arzimanoglou A, Baumgartner C, et al. Classification of paroxysmal events and the four-dimensional epilepsy classification system. Epileptic Disord. 2019;21(1):1–29.
5. Pessin MS, Adelman LS, Prager RJ, Lathi ES, Lange DJ. "Wrong-way eyes" in supratentorial hemorrhage. Ann Neurol. 1981;9(1):79–81.
6. Sharpe JA, Bondar RL, Fletcher WA. Contralateral gaze deviation after frontal lobe haemorrhage. J Neurol Neurosurg Psychiatry. 1985;48(1):86–8.
7. Johkura K, Nakae Y, Yamamoto R, Mitomi M, Kudo Y. Wrong-way deviation: contralateral conjugate eye deviation in acute supratentorial stroke. J Neurol Sci. 2011;308(1-2):165–7.
8. Wu YJ, Tsai TT, Huang CW. Contraversive shift of conjugate eye deviation in hemispheric stroke indicates emerging mass effect. J Clin Neurosci. 2011;18(9):1276–8.
9. Messe SR, Cucchiara BL. Wrong-way eyes with thalamic hemorrhage. Neurology. 2003;60(9):1524.
10. Saiki M, Matsubara T, Suzuki K, Okamura M, Takekawa H, Nakamura T, et al. Conjugate eye deviation due to pontine infarction: report of 2 cases. eNeurologicalSci. 2018;11:1–2.

11. Teufel J, Strupp M, Linn J, Kalla R, Feil K. Conjugate eye deviation in unilateral lateral medullary infarction. J Clin Neurol. 2019;15(2): 228–34.
12. Kobayashi Z, Numasawa Y, Tomimitsu H, Shintani S. Conjugate eye deviation plus spontaneous nystagmus as a diagnostic sign of lateral medullary infarction. J Neurol Sci. 2016;367:222–3.
13. Ogawa T, Ueno Y, Kamo H, Miyamoto N, Yamashiro K, Tanaka R, et al. Conjugate eye deviation caused by upper medial medullary infarction: a case report. J Stroke Cerebrovasc Dis. 2018;27(9):e221–e3.
14. Fisher A, Knezevic W. Ocular and ocular motor aspects of primary thalamic haemorrhage. Clin Exp Neurol. 1985;21:129–39.
15. Choi KD, Jung DS, Kim JS. Specificity of "peering at the tip of the nose" for a diagnosis of thalamic hemorrhage. Arch Neurol. 2004;61(3):417–22.
16. Keane JR, Rawlinson RG, Lu AT. Sustained downgaze deviation. Two cases without structural pretectal lesions. Neurology. 1976;26(6 PT 1):594–5.
17. Johkura K, Komiyama A, Kuroriwa Y. Sustained downgaze in coma after cardiac arrest. J Neurol Neurosurg Psychiatry. 2001;71(2):278–9.
18. Johkura K, Komiyama A, Kuroiwa Y. Vertical conjugate eye deviation in postresuscitation coma. Ann Neurol. 2004;56(6):878–81.
19. Rosenberg ML. The eyes in hysterical states of unconsciousness. J Clin Neuroophthalmol. 1982;2(4):259–60.
20. Keane JR. Sustained upgaze in coma. Ann Neurol. 1981;9(4):409–12.
21. Nakada T, Kwee IL, Lee H. Sustained upgaze in coma. J Clin Neuroophthalmol. 1984;4(1):35–7.
22. Scholz W. Selective neuronal necrosis and its topistic patterns in hypoxemia and oligemia. J Neuropathol Exp Neurol. 1953;12(3):249–61.
23. Adams JH, Brierley JB, Connor RC, Treip CS. The effects of systemic hypotension upon the human brain. Clinical and neuropathological observations in 11 cases. Brain. 1966;89(2):235–68.
24. Leigh RJ, Foley JM, Remler BF, Civil RH. Oculogyric crisis: a syndrome of thought disorder and ocular deviation. Ann Neurol. 1987;22(1):13–7.
25. Tahir H, Daruwalla V. Phencyclidine induced oculogyric crisis responding well to conventional treatment. Case Rep Emerg Med. 2015;2015:506301.
26. Janik P, Figura M. Tetrabenazine-induced oculogyric crisis - a rare complication in the treatment of Gilles de la Tourette syndrome. Neuropsychiatr Dis Treat. 2016;12:497–9.
27. Sarma S, Chetia D, Raha B, Agarwal G. Clozapine withdrawal emergent dystonia, oculogyric crisis and rebound psychosis in a single patient. Ther Adv Psychopharmacol. 2016;6(2):145–6.

28. Barow E, Schneider SA, Bhatia KP, Ganos C. Oculogyric crises: etiology, pathophysiology and therapeutic approaches. Parkinsonism Relat Disord. 2017;36:3–9.
29. Das S, Agrawal A. Lurasidone-induced oculogyric crisis. Indian J Psychol Med. 2017;39(5):719–20.
30. Nebhinani N, Suthar N. Oculogyric crisis with atypical antipsychotics: a case series. Indian J Psychiatry. 2017;59(4):499–501.
31. Wong LH, Tan E. Anti-tuberculosis medication-induced oculogyric crisis and the importance of proper history taking. Int Med Case Rep J. 2017;10:341–4.
32. Davis JL, Kurek JA, Morgan JC, Sethi KD. Teaching video neuroimages: oculogyric crisis in treated Parkinson disease. Neurology. 2018;90(3):e263.
33. Suthar N, Nebhinani N. Aripiprazole induced neck dystonia and oculogyric crisis. Asian J Psychiatr. 2018;31:94–5.
34. Civardi C, Collini A, Geda C. Oculogyric crisis in proton pump inhibitor-associated hypomagnesemia. Parkinsonism Relat Disord. 2020;72:80–1.
35. Keane JR. Spastic eyelids. Failure of levator inhibition in unconscious states. Arch Neurol. 1975;32(10):695–8.
36. Fisher CM. Ocular Bobbing. Arch Neurol. 1964;11:543–6.
37. Hameroff SB, Garcia-Mullin R, Eckholdt J. Ocular bobbing. Arch Ophthalmol. 1969;82(6):774–80.
38. Nelson JR, Johnston CH. Ocular bobbing. Arch Neurol. 1970;22(4): 348–56.
39. Daroff RB. Ocular bobbing. Br Med J. 1971;2(5759):468.
40. Gaymard B. Disconjugate ocular bobbing. Neurology. 1993;43(10):2151.
41. Boddie HG. Ocular bobbing and opsoclonus: two abnormal spontaneous eye movements occurring in the same patient: case report. J Neurol Neurosurg Psychiatry. 1972;35(5):739–42.
42. Paty DW, Sherr H. Ocular bobbing in bromism. A case report. Neurology. 1972;22(5):526–7.
43. Bosch EP, Kennedy SS, Aschenbrener CA. Ocular bobbing: the myth of its localizing value. Neurology. 1975;25(10):949–53.
44. Rai GS, Buxton-Thomas M, Scanlon M. Ocular bobbing in hepatic encephalopathy. Br J Clin Pract. 1976;30(10):202–5.
45. Finelli PF, McEntee WJ. Ocular bobbing with extra-axial haematoma of posterior fossa. J Neurol Neurosurg Psychiatry. 1977;40(4):386–8.
46. Rudick R, Satran R, Eskin TA. Ocular bobbing in encephalitis. J Neurol Neurosurg Psychiatry. 1981;44(5):441–3.
47. Schneider J, Rossetti AO, Alvarez V. Ocular bobbing/dipping after cardiac arrest may be a post-anoxic myoclonus. Resuscitation. 2018;124:e7.
48. Chang TP, Gold DR, Otero-Millan J, Huang BR, Zee DS. Pendular oscillation and ocular bobbing after pontine hemorrhage. Cerebellum.

2019. https://doi.org/10.1007/s12311-019-01086-6. [online ahead of print].
49. Keane JR. Pretectal pseudobobbing. Five patients with 'V'-pattern convergence nystagmus. Arch Neurol. 1985;42(6):592–4.
50. Rosenberg ML, Calvert PC. Ocular bobbing in association with other signs of midbrain dysfunction. Arch Neurol. 1986;43(4):314–5.
51. Noda S, Ide K, Umezaki H, Itoh H, Yamamoto K. Repetitive divergence. Ann Neurol. 1987;21(1):109–10.
52. Das VE, Oruganti P, Kramer PD, Leigh RJ. Experimental tests of a neural-network model for ocular oscillations caused by disease of central myelin. Exp Brain Res. 2000;133(2):189–97.
53. van Weerden TW, van Woerkom TC. Ocular dipping. Clin Neurol Neurosurg. 1982;84(4):221–6.
54. Safran AB, Berney J. Synchronism of reverse ocular bobbing and blinking. Am J Ophthalmol. 1983;95(3):401–2.
55. Haraguchi T, Akaura K, Yabuki S. Creutzfeldt-Jakob disease associated with ocular dipping--a case report. Rinsho Shinkeigaku. 1998;38(1):70–3.
56. Mehler MF. The clinical spectrum of ocular bobbing and ocular dipping. J Neurol Neurosurg Psychiatry. 1988;51(5):725–7.
57. Titer EM, Laureno R. Inverse/reverse ocular bobbing. Ann Neurol. 1988;23(1):103–4.
58. Oh YM, Jeong SH, Kim JS. Ocular dipping and ping-pong gaze in hypoxic encephalopathy. Neurology. 2007;68(3):222.
59. Jeong SH, Kim SY, Park SH, Kim JS. Ocular dipping in Creutzfeldt-Jakob disease. J Neuroophthalmol. 2008;28(4):293–5.
60. Sierra-Hidalgo F, Llamas S, Gonzalo JF, Sanchez Sanchez C. Ocular dipping in creutzfeldt-jakob disease. J Clin Neurol. 2014;10(2):162–5.
61. Lin HJ, Hung TY, Hsieh YJ, Tsai JJ, Huang CW. Spontaneous and stimulus-induced rhythmic periodic or ictal discharges (SIRPIDs) with rhythmic eye blinking and ocular dipping in a post-anoxic comatose patient: a case report. Neurol Sci. 2016;37(12):2027–30.
62. Gray IN, Cristancho AG, Licht DJ, Liu GT. Ocular dipping in a patient with hemiplegic migraine. J Pediatr Ophthalmol Strabismus. 2018;55:e4–6.
63. Jeanneret V, Beach PA, Kase CS. Ocular dipping in anoxic brain injury. JAMA Neurol. 2019;76(10):1252.
64. Rosenberg ML. Spontaneous vertical eye movements in coma. Ann Neurol. 1986;20(5):635–7.
65. Lennox G. Reverse ocular bobbing due to combined phenothiazine and benzodiazepine poisoning. J Neurol Neurosurg Psychiatry. 1993;56(10):1136–7.
66. Cassidy L, Taylor D, Werner K, Veys P, Harris C. Reverse and converse ocular bobbing with synkinetic blinking and opsoclonus in a child with Epstein-Barr virus encephalitis after bone marrow transplant for MPS I. Br J Ophthalmol. 2000;84(10):1207–8.

67. Rehman F, Mehler MF. Reverse ocular dipping. Neurology. 1988;38(3):506.
68. Kuroiwa Y, Toda H. Clinical aspects of abnormal eye movements. Rinsho Shinkeigaku. 2003;43(11):765–8.
69. Kitagawa N, Sakurai M. Drug-induced reverse ocular dipping. BMJ Case Rep. 2014;2014:bcr2014206951.
70. Ishikawa H, Ishikawa S, Mukuno K. Short-cycle periodic alternating (ping-pong) gaze. Neurology. 1993;43(6):1067–70.
71. Yang SL, Han X, Guo CN, Zhu XY, Dong Q, Wang Y. A closer look at ping-pong gaze: an observational study and literature review. J Neurol. 2018;265(12):2825–33.
72. Fisher CM. Some neuro-ophthalmological observations. J Neurol Neurosurg Psychiatry. 1967;30(5):383–92.
73. Reynard M, Wertenbaker C, Behrens M, Lesser R, Eggers H, Ilson J, et al. "Ping-pong gaze" amplified. Neurology. 1979;29(5):757–8.
74. Stewart JD, Kirkham TH, Mathieson G. Periodic alternating gaze. Neurology. 1979;29(2):222–4.
75. Brusa A, Firpo MP, Piccardo A, Stoehr R, Bronzini E. Roving lateral eye movements in coma. A clinical-pathological study. Ital J Neurol Sci. 1984;5(3):279–84.
76. Larmande P, Dongmo L, Limodin J, Ruchoux M. Periodic alternating gaze: a case without any hemispheric lesion. Neurosurgery. 1987;20(3):481–3.
77. Diesing TS, Wijdicks EF. Ping-pong gaze in coma may not indicate persistent hemispheric damage. Neurology. 2004;63(8):1537–8.
78. Gold DR, Aquino KM, Cronin CA. Local(eyes)ing signs in sequential bihemispheric strokes. Neurologist. 2012;18(6):389–90.
79. Moccia M, Allocca R, Erro R, Barone P, Vitale C. Ping-pong gaze: Sherrington would not have done it better. JAMA Neurol. 2014;71(11):1450.
80. Asakura T, Mori N. Roving eye movements in a patient with hypoglycemic coma. Clin Case Rep. 2015;3(5):335–6.
81. Goldberg RT, Gonzalez C, Breinin GM, Reuben RN. Periodic alternating gaze deviation with dissociation of head movement. Arch Ophthalmol. 1965;73:324–30.
82. Senelick RC. "Ping-pong" gaze. Periodic alternating gaze deviation. Neurology. 1976;26(6 PT 1):532–5.
83. Kennard C, Barger G, Hoyt WF. The association of periodic alternating nystagmus with periodic alternating gaze. A case report. J Clin Neuroophthalmol. 1981;1(3):191–3.
84. Grant MP, Cohen M, Petersen RB, Halmagyi GM, McDougall A, Tusa RJ, et al. Abnormal eye movements in Creutzfeldt-Jakob disease. Ann Neurol. 1993;34(2):192–7.
85. Averbuch-Heller L, Meiner Z. Reversible periodic alternating gaze deviation in hepatic encephalopathy. Neurology. 1995;45(1):191–2.

86. Hamed LM, Silbiger J. Periodic alternating esotropia. J Pediatr Ophthalmol Strabismus. 1992;29(4):240–2.
87. Mackay DD, Zepeda Garcia R, Galetta SL, Prasad S. Periodic alternating gaze deviation and nystagmus in posterior reversible encephalopathy syndrome. Neurol Clin Pract. 2014;4(6):482–5.
88. Keane JR, Itabashi HH. Upbeat nystagmus: clinicopathologic study of two patients. Neurology. 1987;37(3):491–4.
89. Munro NA, Gaymard B, Rivaud S, Majdalani A, Pierrot-Deseilligny C. Upbeat nystagmus in a patient with a small medullary infarct. J Neurol Neurosurg Psychiatry. 1993;56(10):1126–8.
90. Hirose G, Ogasawara T, Shirakawa T, Kawada J, Kataoka S, Yoshioka A, et al. Primary position upbeat nystagmus due to unilateral medial medullary infarction. Ann Neurol. 1998;43(3):403–6.
91. Janssen JC, Larner AJ, Morris H, Bronstein AM, Farmer SF. Upbeat nystagmus: clinicoanatomical correlation. J Neurol Neurosurg Psychiatry. 1998;65(3):380–1.
92. Ohkoshi N, Komatsu Y, Mizusawa H, Kanazawa I. Primary position upbeat nystagmus increased on downward gaze: clinicopathologic study of a patient with multiple sclerosis. Neurology. 1998;50(2):551–3.
93. Tilikete C, Hermier M, Pelisson D, Vighetto A. Saccadic lateropulsion and upbeat nystagmus: disorders of caudal medulla. Ann Neurol. 2002;52(5):658–62.
94. Kim JS, Yoon B, Choi KD, Oh SY, Park SH, Kim BK. Upbeat nystagmus: clinicoanatomical correlations in 15 patients. J Clin Neurol. 2006;2(1):58–65.
95. Pierrot-Deseilligny C, Richeh W, Bolgert F. Upbeat nystagmus due to a caudal medullary lesion and influenced by gravity. J Neurol. 2007;254(1):120–1.
96. Saito T, Aizawa H, Sawada J, Katayama T, Hasebe N. Lesion of the nucleus intercalatus in primary position upbeat nystagmus. Arch Neurol. 2010;67(11):1403–4.
97. Adamec I, Gabelic T, Krbot M, Ozretic D, Milivojevic I, Habek M. Primary position upbeat nystagmus. J Clin Neurosci. 2012;19(1):161–2.
98. Troost BT, Martinez J, Abel LA, Heros RC. Upbeat nystagmus and internuclear ophthalmoplegia with brainstem glioma. Arch Neurol. 1980;37(7):453–6.
99. Lee SC, Lee SH, Lee KY, Lee YJ, Koh SH. Transient upbeat nystagmus due to unilateral focal pontine infarction. J Clin Neurosci. 2009;16(4):563–5.
100. Kim JA, Jeong IH, Lim YM, Kim KK. Primary position upbeat nystagmus during an acute attack of multiple sclerosis. J Clin Neurol. 2014;10(1):37–41.
101. Kim HA, Yi HA, Lee H. Can upbeat nystagmus increase in downward, but not upward, gaze? J Clin Neurosci. 2012;19(4):600–1.

102. Kattah JC, Tehrani AS, du Lac S, Newman-Toker DE, Zee DS. Conversion of upbeat to downbeat nystagmus in Wernicke encephalopathy. Neurology. 2018;91(17):790–6.
103. Kattah JC, McClelland C, Zee DS. Vertical nystagmus in Wernicke's encephalopathy: pathogenesis and role of central processing of information from the otoliths. J Neurol. 2019;266(Suppl 1):139–45.
104. Lopez L, Bronstein AM, Gresty MA, Rudge P, du Boulay EP. Torsional nystagmus. A neuro-otological and MRI study of thirty-five cases. Brain. 1992;115(Pt 4):1107–24.
105. Nogues M, Lopez L, Meli F. Neuro-ophthalmologic complications of syringobulbia. Curr Neurol Neurosci Rep. 2010;10(6):459–66.
106. Daroff RB. See-Saw Nystagmus. Neurology. 1965;15:874–7.
107. Nakada T, Kwee IL. Seesaw nystagmus. Role of visuovestibular interaction in its pathogenesis. J Clin Neuroophthalmol. 1988;8(3):171–7.
108. Halmagyi GM, Aw ST, Dehaene I, Curthoys IS, Todd MJ. Jerk-waveform see-saw nystagmus due to unilateral meso-diencephalic lesion. Brain. 1994;117(Pt 4):789–803.
109. Khan SR, Lueck CJ. Hemi-seesaw nystagmus in lateral medullary syndrome. Neurology. 2013;80(13):1261–2.
110. Lee SU, Park SH, Jeong SH, Kim HJ, Kim JS. Evolution of torsional-upbeat into hemi-seesaw nystagmus in medial medullary infarction. Clin Neurol Neurosurg. 2014;118:80–2.
111. Yunusov F, Park JH, Huh YE, Kim HJ, Kim JS. Mystery case: pendular see-saw nystagmus as a delayed complication of traumatic brain injury. Neurology. 2014;82(17):e147–8.
112. Hari Kumar KVS, Singh P. Seesaw Nystagmus. N Engl J Med. 2017;376(24):e51.
113. Lee H, Kim HA. Hemi-seesaw nystagmus in a patient with acute infarction in the superior cerebellar artery territory. J Neurol. 2018;265(5):1219–21.
114. Drachman DA. See-saw nystagmus. J Neurol Neurosurg Psychiatry. 1966;29(4):356–61.
115. Bergin DJ, Halpern J. Congenital see-saw nystagmus associated with retinitis pigmentosa. Ann Ophthalmol. 1986;18(12):346–9.
116. May EF, Truxal AR. Loss of vision alone may result in seesaw nystagmus. J Neuroophthalmol. 1997;17(2):84–5.
117. Jeong SH, Hwang JM, Kim JS. Co-occurrence of periodic alternating and pendular seesaw nystagmus in blindness. J Neurol Sci. 2009;285(1-2):257–8.
118. Choi KD, Jung DS, Park KP, Jo JW, Kim JS. Bowtie and upbeat nystagmus evolving into hemi-seesaw nystagmus in medial medullary infarction: possible anatomic mechanisms. Neurology. 2004;62(4):663–5.
119. Choi SY, Kim DH, Lee JH, Kim J. Jerky hemi-seesaw nystagmus and head tilt reaction combined with internuclear ophthalmoplegia from a pontine infarction. J Clin Neurosci. 2009;16(3):456–8.

120. Rosenberg M, Sharpe J, Hoyt WF. Absent vestibulo-ocular reflexes and acute supratentorial lesions. J Neurol Neurosurg Psychiatry. 1975;38(1): 6–10.
121. Hanid MA, Silk DB, Williams R. Prognostic value of the oculovestibular reflex in fulminant hepatic failure. Br Med J. 1978;1(6119):1029.
122. Keane JR. Acute bilateral ophthalmoplegia: 60 cases. Neurology. 1986;36(2):279–81.
123. Uematsu D, Suematsu M, Fukuuchi Y, Ebihara S, Gotoh F. Midbrain locked-in state with oculomotor subnucleus lesion. J Neurol Neurosurg Psychiatry. 1985;48(9):952–3.
124. Caplan LR, Scheiner D. Dysconjugate gaze in hepatic coma. Ann Neurol. 1980;8(3):328–9.
125. Cook FF, Davis RG, Russo LS Jr. Internuclear ophthalmoplegia caused by phenothiazine intoxication. Arch Neurol. 1981;38(7):465–6.
126. Hotson JR, Sachdev HS. Amitriptyline: another cause of internuclear ophthalmoplegia with coma. Ann Neurol. 1982;12(1):62.
127. Rizzo M, Corbett J. Bilateral internuclear ophthalmoplegia reversed by naloxone. Arch Neurol. 1983;40(4):242–3.
128. Donhowe SP. Bilateral internuclear ophthalmoplegia from doxepin overdose. Neurology. 1984;34(2):259.
129. el-Mallakh RS. Internuclear ophthalmoplegia with narcotic overdosage. Ann Neurol. 1986;20(1):107.
130. Simon RP. Forced downward ocular deviation. Occurrence during oculovestibular testing in sedative drug-induced coma. Arch Neurol. 1978;35(7):456–8.
131. Singh BM, Strobos RJ. Retraction nystagmus elicited by bilateral simultaneous cold caloric stimulation. Ann Neurol. 1980;8(1):79.

Eye Movements and Vestibular Dysfunction: Lesions of Medulla Oblongata

6

Medulla oblongata, the caudal most part of the brainstem, houses several nuclei and pathways that are pivotal for the eye movements. Medullary lesions can cause a range of eye movement abnormalities. This chapter summarizes the ocular motor manifestations of the structural deficits in medulla oblongata that are seen in critical care setting.

Acute Vestibular Syndrome

Acute vestibular syndrome is one of the most common ways the medullary lesions present in the acute care settings, in the emergency rooms and in the critical care units. The deficits are typically characterized by acute onset of vertigo that is intractable and is associated with nausea, vomiting, and unsteady gait [1, 2]. Although typical etiology is peripheral end-organ dysfunction such as the vestibular neuritis, the central causes are also likely [1]. The ischemic events involving the brainstem or the cerebellum also cause the acute vestibular syndrome in about 10% of the patients [3]. Medullary etiologies of the acute vestibular syndrome are discussed here, the other causes of the acute vestibular syndrome are discussed in their respective chapters. The lateral medullary syndrome, also known as the Wallenberg's syndrome, is the common cause of acute vestibular syndrome due to the medullary etiologies [4–12].

A. Shaikh, F. Wang, *Eye Movements in the Critical Care Setting*,
https://doi.org/10.1007/978-3-030-70221-2_6

Lateral Medullary Syndrome (Wallenberg's Syndrome)

The lateral medullary syndrome, also known as the Wallenberg's syndrome, is associated with the lesions affecting the lateral medulla and the inferior cerebellar peduncle projecting to the inferolateral cerebellum. Each of these anatomical areas corresponds with the specific eye movement deficit seen in the lateral medullary syndrome.

Lateropulsion is associated with the lesion affecting the inferior cerebellar peduncle that houses the climbing fibers from the contralateral inferior olive nucleus. The deficit characterized by the tonic lateral deviation of the eyes is typically prominent under the closed eyelids (Fig. 6.1). Figure 6.1 depicts the simplified explanation of lateropulsion. The contralateral inferior olive sends inhibitory climbing fibers through inferior cerebellar peduncle (ICP) to reach the dorsal vermis. Dorsal vermis then inhibits the fastigial ocular region (FOR). Lesion involving the ICP leads to inhibition of the ipsilateral FOR. Imbalance between two FORs lead to ipsilateral deviation of the eyes during lid closure (i.e., lateropulsion) or during saccades (i.e., ipsipulsion). Lateropulsion is identified while looking for the horizontal deviation of the eyes (the corneal bulge under closed eye lids) when the eyelids are closed [13–15]. Lateropulsion could also be identified when the patient stares at the target straight-ahead, then transiently closes the eyelids or blinks, after eyelids open there would be a corrective saccade to bring the eyes back to center. However, in severe cases, conjugate gaze deviation from lateropulsion could occur even with the eyes open [16]. Lateropulsion could also affect saccades [13, 15]. Such deficit is called ipsipulsion, where the horizontal saccades towards the lesion sides are hypermetric, whereas the saccades directed away from the lesion are hypometric [13, 17, 18]. Furthermore, the quick phase of nystagmus, sharing the same physiological mechanism as saccades, is also affected in lateropulsion. The quick phase directed away from the lesion have relatively smaller amplitude compared to the one towards the lesion. In some cases, lateropulsion also modifies the trajectory of

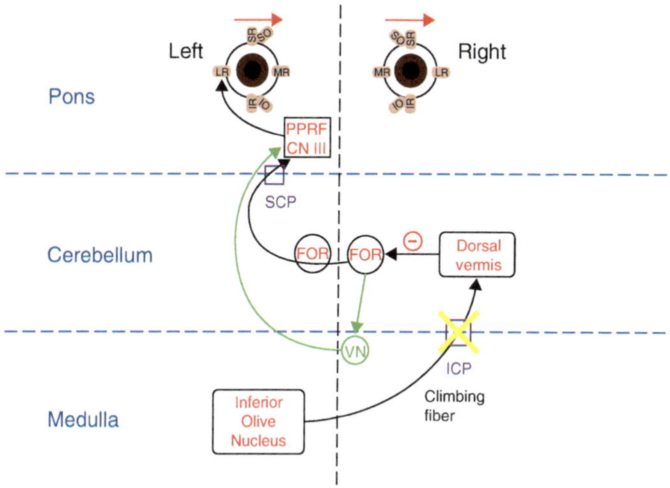

Fig. 6.1 A diagrammatic illustration of the mechanism for lateropulsion and ipsipulsion. The inferior olive nucleus normally inhibits the contralateral dorsal vermis of cerebellum via contralateral inferior cerebellar peduncle (ICP). As depicted here, the right Wallenberg's syndrome affects the right-sided ICP which causes the disinhibition of the ipsilateral dorsal vermis of cerebellum. Such disinhibition then leads to the imbalance between bilateral fastigial nuclei (FOR) with the dominance on the left side. Thus, the eyes are pushed to the right during eyelid closure, or there is rightward deviation of open eyes in those with severe impairment. The same mechanism also accounts for curvature of the vertical saccades towards the affected side. The FOR acts as brakes leading to saccade termination. Because of such imbalance between the FORs, the right-ward saccades overshoot and left-ward saccades undershoot. As a result hypermetric saccades are seen towards right side and hypometric saccades towards left side in right-sided Wallenberg's syndrome

vertical eye movements. Vertical movements deviate towards the side of the lesion followed by the correction to the midline causing curved vertical saccade trajectory with the convexity towards the lesion [19, 20].

Ocular tilt reaction is secondary to the involvement of medullary graviceptive pathways involving the vestibular nucleus and its connections (Fig. 6.2). Figure 6.2 illustrates simplified graviceptive pathway. The utricle, sensing gravity and head tilt, sends

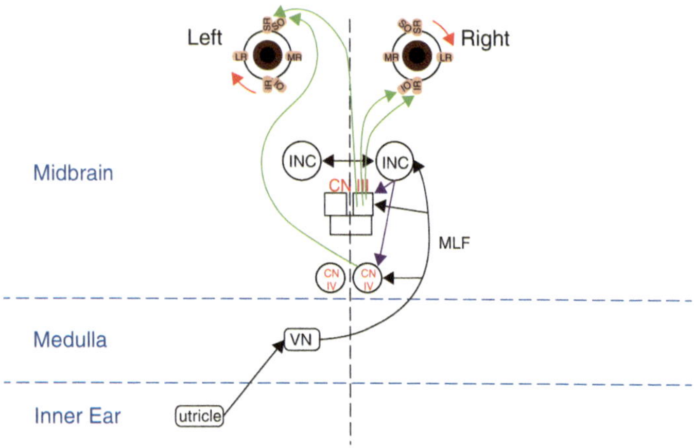

Fig. 6.2 A schematic depicting the mechanism of ocular tilt reaction. The involvement of vestibular nucleus in Wallenberg's syndrome causes the imbalance of bilateral utricular input. In the setting of right-sided Wallenberg's syndrome, the left vestibular nucleus dominates, and the brain perceives it as the right ear is tilting to the right shoulder. Thus, via the connections of medial longitudinal fasciculus, the right eye extorts and depresses, the left eye intorts and elevates, and the head tilts towards left to "compensate" the perceived tilt

the signal to the vestibular nucleus which then moves the eyes through the cranial nerve III and IV. Lesion involving one utricle lead to input signal imbalance leading to ocular tilt reaction. The constellation of impairments include misperception of visual verticality (subjective visual vertical), tonic torsional rotation of the eyes, skew deviation, and compensatory head or body tilt [21–23]. The impaired percept of verticality leads to the sensation as if the floor is ending on the ceiling [13]. It is also possible to have an incomplete ocular tilt reaction. Imbalance in utricular input leads to upward deviation of the contralateral eye [24, 25]. The ipsilateral eye may stay put if the projections from the same side are spared.

Spontaneous nystagmus in lateral medullary syndrome is typically pure horizontal or torsional with horizontal and vertical components [26]. When it is horizontal, it typically has quick phase directed opposite to side of the lesion, the torsional quick

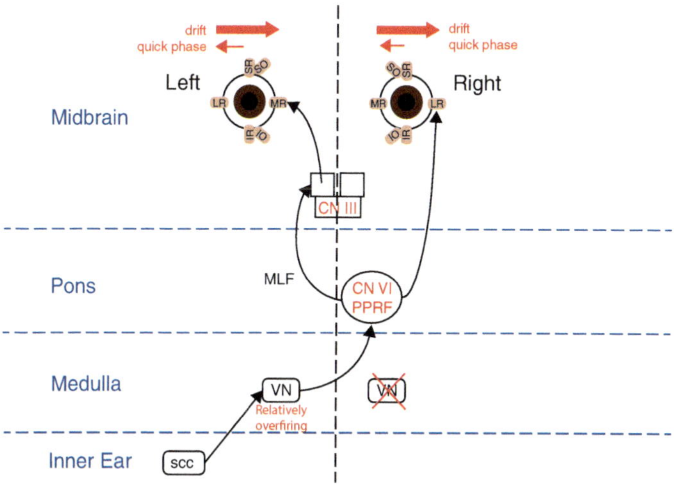

Fig. 6.3 The diagram demonstrates a pathway for horizontal nystagmus. Illustrated lesion on the right vestibular nucleus (VN) leads to imbalance of inputs from both sides. The "hyperactive" left VN drives both eyes towards right side and then rapid corrective saccades beating to the left

phase is in the direction towards the lesion [13, 26–29] (Fig. 6.3). The Figure 6.3 demonstrates the neuronal basis for the generation of horizontal nystagmus. The lesion involving the vestibular nucleus on one side leads to imbalance of the vestibular inputs, which drifts the eyes towards the lesion side. With intact visual system the eyes rapidly return with corrective saccades, i.e., the quick phase of nystagmus [28]. It is also possible to have vestibular nystagmus mixed with the gaze-evoked nystagmus. The nystagmus at the onset of active or passive head-shaking side-by-side (head-shaking nystagmus) can be present; in such cases the direction of quick phase are towards the side of the lesion [29]. Hemi-seesaw nystagmus, jerk-waveform nystagmus with conjugate torsional and disjunctive vertical components, can be seen in those with Wallenberg's syndrome [26, 30–32].

Smooth pursuit is usually impaired in the lateral medullary syndrome. Characteristically tracking the targets moving towards the side contralateral to the lesion is most affected [33, 34].

Other ocular motor abnormalities in lateral medullary syndrome include hypoactive caloric response on the side of the lesion. Such deficits are most likely when the vestibular nucleus is involved. The caudal medullary lesions in the Wallenberg's syndrome can also cause delayed cervical vestibular-evoked myogenic potentials (c-VEMPS), a physiological correlate that determines vestibular function by applying a repetitive sound stimulus to one ear and then averaging the reaction of the cervical muscle activity in response to each sound click or pulse [35].

The ocular motor abnormalities seen in the lateral medullary syndrome is outline in Table 6.1.

The lateral medullary syndrome can also have other, non-ocular motor or vestibular, presentations [36–41]. Ipsilateral impairment of pain and temperature sensation over the face via involvement of the trigeminal tract is well described in this condition. Ipsilateral Horner's syndrome (secondary to the involvement of sympathetic pathway) is also expected. Ipsilateral limb ataxia is common, and it is due to involvement of the inferior cerebellar peduncle. Bulbar symptoms and lower motor neuron facial paresis are reported. Abnormal hiccups are characteristic sign of the lesion involving the area postrema [39, 40].

Table 6.1 Ocular motor dysfunctions of Wallenberg's syndrome [42]

Lateropulsion (Deviation) of the eyes toward side of the lesion occurs in darkness, behind closed lids or with a blink
Lateropulsion (Ipsipulsion) of horizontal saccades: ipsilateral (toward the lesion side) saccades are hypermetric, contralateral are hypometric
Lateropulsion of vertical saccades causing an oblique trajectory
Torsipulsion: Inappropriate torsional deviations may occur during horizontal saccades
Smooth pursuit is impaired for targets moving **away** from the side of lesion
Spontaneous nystagmus (often mixed horizontal and torsional) occurs with the eyes in central position; slow phase may be directed towards or away from the side of the lesion
Ocular tilt reaction (OTR): skew deviation with ipsilateral hypo-deviation, head tilt towards side of the lesion, ipsilateral cyclodeviation; ipsilateral deviation of subjective visual vertical

Medial Medullary Syndrome

Several nuclei responsible for the control of eye movements reside in the medial medulla. Nucleus prepositus hypoglossi (NPH), in the floor of fourth ventricle, together with nucleus of Roller and caudal nucleus of intercalatus of Staderini form the perihypoglossal nuclei [43]. Neurons in the NPH and adjacent medial vestibular nuclei (MVN) are known to be the neural integrators for horizontal eccentric gaze holding [44]. Other paramedian medullary structures that contribute to the normal gaze holding are the cell groups of paramedian tracts (PMT) which include six groups of neurons spreading out in the paramedian structure of the entire brainstem. They relay information from premotor nuclei concerned with eye movements to the vestibulocerebellum [43, 45].

The typical deficit due to acute lesions of paramedian medullary structures is gaze-evoked nystagmus in combination with the postural imbalance and vertigo. The impairments are secondary to the involvement of the neural integrator [46–48]. Paramedian medullary lesions are also known to cause several forms of jerk nystagmus when the eyes are in primary gaze, for example upbeat, downbeat, torsional and hemi-seesaw (Fig. 6.4).

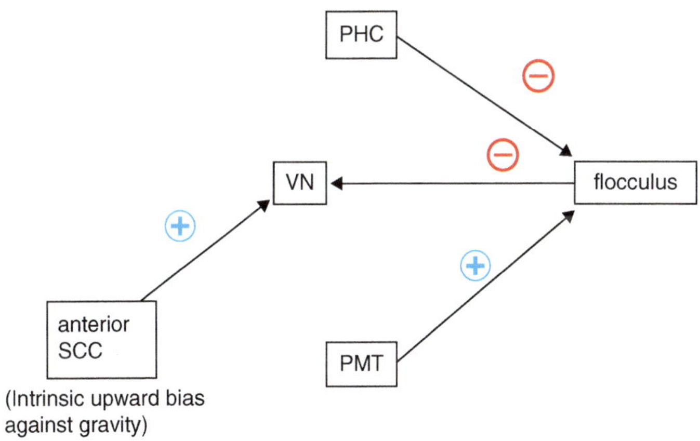

Fig. 6.4 A simplified schematic depicts a network between nuclei in the median medulla and cerebellum

The Figure 6.4 depicts the simplified connections scheme between the paramedian medullary nuclei and the cerebellum for better understanding of the generation of different forms of nystagmus. The upbeat nystagmus is common in paramedian medullary syndrome [49–54]. Normally there is an intrinsic upward bias against gravity to maintain eye position while we are standing. Lesions involving the ascending vestibular pathways, for example the crossing ventral tegmental pathway, lead to the downward eyes drift with a rapid upward correction [49, 55–59]. The lesion of NPH which normally inhibits the floccular complexes in the cerebellum can also lead to up-down imbalance in the vestibular nucleus, subsequently leading to downward drift and upward quick phase [60]. The upbeat-torsional nystagmus that is occasionally seen with the medial medullary syndrome can be due to the involvement of the anterior semicircular canal axons in the medulla. The hemi-seesaw nystagmus is seen if such lesion progresses to involve both anterior and posterior semicircular canals [57, 61]. Involvement of PMT could lead to downbeat nystagmus [62–64]. If upbeat nystagmus is associated with bilateral internuclear ophthalmoplegia usually indicates the involvement of PMT cell groups [65]. Paramedian medullary lesion can also lead to ocular tilt reaction, this is due to the involvement of the graviceptive pathways crossing over at the level of pontomedullary junction [32]. Furthermore, contrapulsion of saccades can be seen if the climbing fiber from ipsilateral inferior olivary nucleus are affected before they cross the midline (Fig. 6.1) [66].

The medial medullary syndrome typically manifests as contralateral hemiparesis and impaired proprioception (Fig. 6.5). The Figure 6.5 demonstrates the anatomical structures commonly involved in medial medullary syndrome; they include the pyramids, medial lemniscus and fascicles of hypoglossal nerve. The anatomical location of the lesion (such as an infarct) also determines the presence or lateralization of the tongue weakness. The rostral lesion leads to contralateral tongue deviation; whereas the caudal lesion cause ipsilateral tongue deviation [32, 67].

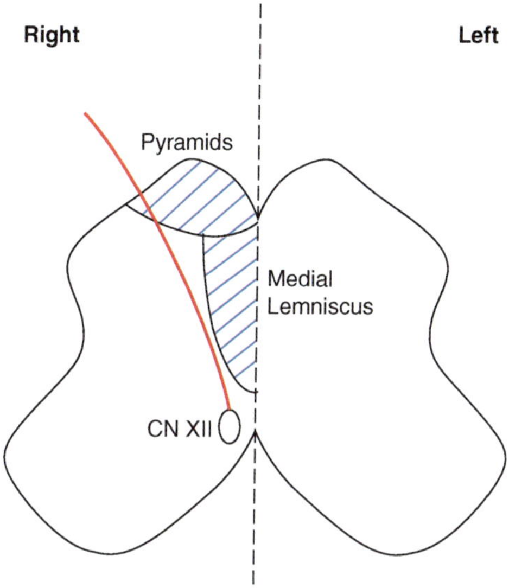

Fig. 6.5 The figure demonstrated right medial medullary syndrome. The involvement of pyramids causes contralateral body hemiparesis or hemiplegia. Injury of medial lemniscus leads to loss of contralateral hemibody deep sensation. Depending on the level of involvement, more rostral lesion damages the corticobulbar tract, which leads to tongue deviation to contralateral side, whereas caudal lesion damages the hypoglossal nerve itself and leads to ipsilateral tongue deviation.

Other Medullary Lesions

Syringobulbia, a late complication of syringomyelia, is due to the upward extension of the syrinx involving the midline structures and their connections. The patients can often have nystagmus, typically torsional with the top pole of eyes beating toward more affected side [68]. Presence of horizontal nystagmus indicates further rostral extension of the syrinx affecting the NPH. Whereas vertical nystagmus, especially upbeat nystagmus suggests involvement of NPH or PMT nuclei. Downbeat nystagmus and seesaw nystagmus can also be seen in the rare occasions, but the mechanism is less clear; one possibility to be considered is the coexistence of the Chiari malformation which is known to cause downbeat as well as seesaw nystagmus [69, 70].

Lacunar infarct is extremely rare in medulla oblongata and most commonly involves in the anterolateral or anteromedial areas of medulla [71]. Isolated NPH lesion has been reported previously, it causes primary gaze upbeat nystagmus with velocity-decreasing slow phase suggesting leaky neural integration [47, 48, 51, 54]. Conjugate gaze deviation to contralateral side was also reported in lesion of NPH secondary to interruption of NPH-inferior olivary nucleus-flocculus-vestibular nucleus loop [72].

Summary

In this chapter, we reviewed the important role of medulla oblongata possesses in eye movements. Acute vestibular syndrome is one of the common presentations that brings patients to the emergency room. It is important to differentiate the central versus peripheral causes. In Wallenberg syndrome (lateral medullary syndrome), there are multiple ocular motor abnormalities can be observed – ipsipulsion, hypermetric saccades, ocular tilt reaction, spontaneous nystagmus and impaired smooth pursuit. Medial medullary syndrome, typically presenting with contralateral hemiparesis and ipsilateral tongue deviation, can also have some eye movement abnormalities. The characteristic one is gaze-evoked nystagmus. Upbeat nystagmus can also be observed at times. Other medullary lesions, such as syringobulbia can present with different types of nystagmus depending on the extent of the lesion.

References

1. Tarnutzer AA, Berkowitz AL, Robinson KA, Hsieh YH, Newman-Toker DE. Does my dizzy patient have a stroke? A systematic review of bedside diagnosis in acute vestibular syndrome. CMAJ. 2011;183(9):E571–92.
2. Hotson JR, Baloh RW. Acute vestibular syndrome. N Engl J Med. 1998;339(10):680–5.

3. Newman-Toker DE. Missed stroke in acute vertigo and dizziness: it is time for action, not debate. Ann Neurol. 2016;79(1):27–31.
4. Estanol B, Lopez-Rios G. Neuro-otology of the lateral medullary infarct syndrome. Arch Neurol. 1982;39(3):176–9.
5. Dieterich M, Brandt T. Imaging cortical activity after vestibular lesions. Restor Neurol Neurosci. 2010;28(1):47–56.
6. Kim MB, Boo SH, Ban JH. Nystagmus-based approach to vertebrobasilar stroke presenting as vertigo without initial neurologic signs. Eur Neurol. 2013;70(5–6):322–8.
7. Saber Tehrani AS, Kattah JC, Mantokoudis G, Pula JH, Nair D, Blitz A, et al. Small strokes causing severe vertigo: frequency of false-negative MRIs and nonlacunar mechanisms. Neurology. 2014;83(2):169–73.
8. Choi JH, Kim HW, Choi KD, Kim MJ, Choi YR, Cho HJ, et al. Isolated vestibular syndrome in posterior circulation stroke: frequency and involved structures. Neurol Clin Pract. 2014;4(5):410–8.
9. Lee SU, Park SH, Park JJ, Kim HJ, Han MK, Bae HJ, et al. Dorsal medullary infarction: distinct syndrome of isolated central vestibulopathy. Stroke. 2015;46(11):3081–7.
10. Ehresmann AM, Van HC, Merlini L, Fluss J. Wallenberg syndrome: an exceptional cause of acute Vertigo in children. Neuropediatrics. 2016;47(1):61–3.
11. Kim HJ, Kim S, Park JH, Kim JS. Altered processing of otolithic information in isolated lateral medullary infarction. J Neurol. 2016;263(12):2424–9.
12. Kattah JC, Saber Tehrani AS, Roeber S, Gujrati M, Bach SE, Newman Toker DE, et al. Transient Vestibulopathy in Wallenberg's syndrome: pathologic analysis. Front Neurol. 2017;8:191.
13. Brazis PW. Ocular motor abnormalities in Wallenberg's lateral medullary syndrome. Mayo Clin Proc. 1992;67(4):365–8.
14. Hornsten G. Wallenberg's syndrome. II. Oculomotor and oculostatic disturbances. Acta Neurol Scand. 1974;50(4):447–68.
15. Kommerell G, Hoyt WF. Lateropulsion of saccadic eye movements. Electro-oculographic studies in a patient with Wallenberg's syndrome. Arch Neurol. 1973;28(5):313–8.
16. Kobayashi Z, Numasawa Y, Tomimitsu H, Shintani S. Conjugate eye deviation plus spontaneous nystagmus as a diagnostic sign of lateral medullary infarction. J Neurol Sci. 2016;367:222–3.
17. Meyer KT, Baloh RW, Krohel GB, Hepler RS. Ocular lateropulsion. A sign of lateral medullary disease. Arch Ophthalmol. 1980;98(9):1614–6.
18. Islam N, Plant GT, Acheson JF. Saccadic lateropulsion or ipsipulsion. Acta Ophthalmol. 2008;86(6):688–9.
19. Kirkham TH, Guitton D, Gans M. Task dependent variations of ocular lateropulsion in Wallenberg's syndrome. Can J Neurol Sci. 1981;8(1):21–6.
20. Kaski D, Bentley P, Lane R, Bronstein A. Up-down asymmetry of saccadic contrapulsion in lateral medullary syndrome. J Neuroophthalmol. 2012;32(3):224–6.

21. Dieterich M, Brandt T. Wallenberg's syndrome: lateropulsion, cyclorotation, and subjective visual vertical in thirty-six patients. Ann Neurol. 1992;31(4):399–408.
22. Brandt T, Dieterich M. Skew deviation with ocular torsion: a vestibular brainstem sign of topographic diagnostic value. Ann Neurol. 1993;33(5):528–34.
23. Brandt T, Dieterich M. Pathological eye-head coordination in roll: tonic ocular tilt reaction in mesencephalic and medullary lesions. Brain. 1987;110(Pt 3):649–66.
24. Brandt TH, Dieterich M. Different types of skew deviation. J Neurol Neurosurg Psychiatry. 1991;54(6):549–50.
25. Brodsky MC, Donahue SP, Vaphiades M, Brandt T. Skew deviation revisited. Surv Ophthalmol. 2006;51(2):105–28.
26. Morrow MJ, Sharpe JA. Torsional nystagmus in the lateral medullary syndrome. Ann Neurol. 1988;24(3):390–8.
27. Tseng CH, Chiu WY. Isolated rotational nystagmus may be the only clue to the early diagnosis of dorsolateral medullary infarction. Am J Emerg Med. 2014;32(7):813 e3–4.
28. Rambold H, Helmchen C. Spontaneous nystagmus in dorsolateral medullary infarction indicates vestibular semicircular canal imbalance. J Neurol Neurosurg Psychiatry. 2005;76(1):88–94.
29. Choi KD, Oh SY, Park SH, Kim JH, Koo JW, Kim JS. Head-shaking nystagmus in lateral medullary infarction: patterns and possible mechanisms. Neurology. 2007;68(17):1337–44.
30. Khan SR, Lueck CJ. Hemi-seesaw nystagmus in lateral medullary syndrome. Neurology. 2013;80(13):1261–2.
31. Porta-Etessam J, Casanova I, Pajuelo B, Di Capua D, del Val J, Garcia ME, et al. See-saw nystagmus in a patient with Wallenberg syndrome. J Neuroophthalmol. 2009;29(1):73–4.
32. Kim JS, Choi KD, Oh SY, Park SH, Han MK, Yoon BW, et al. Medial medullary infarction: abnormal ocular motor findings. Neurology. 2005;65(8):1294–8.
33. Baloh RW, Yee RD, Honrubia V. Eye movements in patients with Wallenberg's syndrome. Ann N Y Acad Sci. 1981;374:600–13.
34. Waespe W, Wichmann W. Oculomotor disturbances during visual-vestibular interaction in Wallenberg's lateral medullary syndrome. Brain. 1990;113(Pt 3):821–46.
35. Tseng CL, Young YH. Topographical correlations of lateral medullary infarction with caloric- and vestibular-evoked myogenic potential results. Eur Arch Otorhinolaryngol. 2010;267(2):191–5.
36. Savitz SI, Caplan LR. Vertebrobasilar disease. N Engl J Med. 2005;352(25):2618–26.
37. Eggers C, Fink GR, Moller-Hartmann W, Nowak DA. Correlation of anatomy and function in medulla oblongata infarction. Eur J Neurol. 2009;16(2):201–4.

38. Moncayo J, Bogousslavsky J. Vertebro-basilar syndromes causing oculomotor disorders. Curr Opin Neurol. 2003;16(1):45–50.
39. Park MH, Kim BJ, Koh SB, Park MK, Park KW, Lee DH. Lesional location of lateral medullary infarction presenting hiccups (singultus). J Neurol Neurosurg Psychiatry. 2005;76(1):95–8.
40. Mandala M, Rufa A, Cerase A, Bracco S, Galluzzi P, Venturi C, et al. Lateral medullary ischemia presenting with persistent hiccups and vertigo. Int J Neurosci. 2010;120(3):226–30.
41. Kim JS. Pure lateral medullary infarction: clinical-radiological correlation of 130 acute, consecutive patients. Brain. 2003;126(Pt 8):1864–72.
42. Leigh RJ, Zee DS. The neurology of eye movements. 5th ed. Oxford ; New York: Oxford University Press; 2015. xx, 1109 pages p
43. Buttner-Ennever JA, Horn AKE, Olszewski J. Olszewski and Baxter's Cytoarchitecture of the human brainstem. 3rd, revised and extended ed. Basel/New York: Karger; 2014. xii, 290 pages p
44. Sanchez K, Rowe FJ. Role of neural integrators in oculomotor systems: a systematic narrative literature review. Acta Ophthalmol. 2018;96(2): e111–e8.
45. Buttner-Ennever JA, Horn AK. Pathways from cell groups of the paramedian tracts to the floccular region. Ann N Y Acad Sci. 1996;781:532–40.
46. Anagnostou E, Spengos K, Margeti S, Vassilopoulou S, Paraskevas GP, Zis V. Vertical and horizontal integrator failure in a ponto-medullary infarction: a possible role for paramedian tract neurons. J Neurol Sci. 2009;280(1–2):118–9.
47. Cho HJ, Choi HY, Kim YD, Seo SW, Heo JH. The clinical syndrome and etiological mechanism of infarction involving the nucleus prepositus hypoglossi. Cerebrovasc Dis. 2008;26(2):178–83.
48. Seo SW, Shin HY, Kim SH, Han SW, Lee KY, Kim SM, et al. Vestibular imbalance associated with a lesion in the nucleus prepositus hypoglossi area. Arch Neurol. 2004;61(9):1440–3.
49. Kim JA, Jeong IH, Lim YM, Kim KK. Primary position upbeat nystagmus during an acute attack of multiple sclerosis. J Clin Neurol. 2014;10(1):37–41.
50. Kim JS, Yoon B, Choi KD, Oh SY, Park SH, Kim BK. Upbeat nystagmus: clinicoanatomical correlations in 15 patients. J Clin Neurol. 2006;2(1): 58–65.
51. Hirose G, Ogasawara T, Shirakawa T, Kawada J, Kataoka S, Yoshioka A, et al. Primary position upbeat nystagmus due to unilateral medial medullary infarction. Ann Neurol. 1998;43(3):403–6.
52. Keane JR, Itabashi HH. Upbeat nystagmus: clinicopathologic study of two patients. Neurology. 1987;37(3):491–4.
53. Saito T, Aizawa H, Sawada J, Katayama T, Hasebe N. Lesion of the nucleus intercalatus in primary position upbeat nystagmus. Arch Neurol. 2010;67(11):1403–4.

54. Ohkoshi N, Komatsu Y, Mizusawa H, Kanazawa I. Primary position upbeat nystagmus increased on downward gaze: clinicopathologic study of a patient with multiple sclerosis. Neurology. 1998;50(2):551–3.
55. Ranalli PJ, Sharpe JA. Upbeat nystagmus and the ventral tegmental pathway of the upward vestibulo-ocular reflex. Neurology. 1988;38(8): 1329–30.
56. Tilikete C, Milea D, Pierrot-Deseilligny C. Upbeat nystagmus from a demyelinating lesion in the caudal pons. J Neuroophthalmol. 2008;28(3): 202–6.
57. Thurtell MJ, Tomsak RL, Leigh RJ. Upbeat-torsional nystagmus and contralateral fourth-nerve palsy due to unilateral dorsal ponto mesencephalic lesion. Ann N Y Acad Sci. 2009;1164:476–8.
58. Nakada T, Remler MP. Primary position upbeat nystagmus. Another central vestibular nystagmus? J Clin Neuroophthalmol. 1981;1(3):185–9.
59. Choi KD, Jung DS, Park KP, Jo JW, Kim JS. Bowtie and upbeat nystagmus evolving into hemi-seesaw nystagmus in medial medullary infarction: possible anatomic mechanisms. Neurology. 2004;62(4):663–5.
60. Kattah JC, Tehrani AS, du Lac S, Newman-Toker DE, Zee DS. Conversion of upbeat to downbeat nystagmus in Wernicke encephalopathy. Neurology. 2018;91(17):790–6.
61. Lee SU, Park SH, Jeong SH, Kim HJ, Kim JS. Evolution of torsional-upbeat into hemi-seesaw nystagmus in medial medullary infarction. Clin Neurol Neurosurg. 2014;118:80–2.
62. Helmchen C, Glasauer S, Sprenger A. Inverse eye position dependency of downbeat nystagmus in midline medullary lesion. J Neurol. 2013;260(11):2908–10.
63. Pierrot-Deseilligny C, Milea D. Vertical nystagmus: clinical facts and hypotheses. Brain. 2005;128(Pt 6):1237–46.
64. Nakamagoe K, Shimizu K, Koganezawa T, Tamaoka A. Downbeat nystagmus due to a paramedian medullary lesion. J Clin Neurosci. 2012;19(11):1597–9.
65. Choi JH, Jung NY, Kim MJ, Choi KD, Kim JS, Jung DS. Pure upbeat nystagmus in association with bilateral internuclear ophthalmoplegia. J Neurol Sci. 2012;317(1–2):148–50.
66. Kim JS, Moon SY, Kim KY, Kim HC, Park SH, Yoon BW, et al. Ocular contrapulsion in rostral medial medullary infarction. Neurology. 2004;63(7):1325–7.
67. Kim JS, Han YS. Medial medullary infarction: clinical, imaging, and outcome study in 86 consecutive patients. Stroke. 2009;40(10):3221–5.
68. Nogues M, Lopez L, Meli F. Neuro-ophthalmologic complications of syringobulbia. Curr Neurol Neurosci Rep. 2010;10(6):459–66.
69. Pinel JF, Larmande P, Guegan Y, Iba-Zizen MT. Down-beat nystagmus: case report with magnetic resonance imaging and surgical treatment. Neurosurgery. 1987;21(5):736–9.

70. Weissman JD, Seidman SH, Dell'osso LF, Naheedy MH, Leigh RJ. Torsional, see-saw, 'bow-tie' nystagmus in association with brain stem anomalies. Neuro-Ophthalmology. 1990;10(6):315–8.
71. Kim K, Lee HS, Jung YH, Kim YD, Nam HS, Nam CM, et al. Mechanism of medullary infarction based on arterial territory involvement. J Clin Neurol. 2012;8(2):116–22.
72. Ogawa T, Ueno Y, Kamo H, Miyamoto N, Yamashiro K, Tanaka R, et al. Conjugate eye deviation caused by upper medial medullary infarction: a case report. J Stroke Cerebrovasc Dis. 2018;27(9):e221–e3.

Eye Movements and Vestibular Dysfunction: Lesions of Cerebellum

7

The cerebellum, located dorsal to the brainstem, has critical role in movement coordination by utilizing two key principles, adapting for unexpected errors and incorporating the anticipated future changes in ongoing movements based on the previous experiences. Study of eye movements have tremendously facilitated our understanding of predictive and adaptive functions of the cerebellum. These principles, tied with anatomically discrete roles of various parts of the cerebellum, put it in the strategic position to facilitate clinical localization. The effects of cerebellar lesions can be classified in three major categories: [1] the syndrome of flocculus and paraflocculus [2], the syndrome of the nodulus and ventral uvula and [3], the syndrome of dorsal vermis and the underlying fastigial nuclei, the fastigial oculomotor region (FOR). Despite theoretical segregation, there is substantial overlap as disease frequently involves more than one functional region of the cerebellum. The functional anatomy of the cerebellum can be instrumental in accurate bedside diagnoses of the critical illnesses such as acute cerebellar strokes. The eye movement examination in these patients can be instrumental in accurate localization within the cerebellar regions. Such skillset is often necessary due to logistic difficulties in obtaining high-resolution posterior fossa imaging in critically ill patients to evaluate for lesions. This chapter has simplified schemes outlining the patterns of abnormal eye movements in patients with various forms of cerebellar lesions.

A. Shaikh, F. Wang, *Eye Movements in the Critical Care Setting*,
https://doi.org/10.1007/978-3-030-70221-2_7

Lesions of Flocculus and Paraflocculus

In animal studies, experimental lesions of flocculus and paraflocculus cause gaze-holding deficits including gaze-evoked nystagmus, rebound nystagmus, downbeat nystagmus and impaired smooth pursuit. All these findings are commonly seen in patients with cerebellar diseases [1]. Pharmaceutical inactivation of flocculus-paraflocculus with muscimol severely impairs smooth pursuit when tracking with the eyes only, however active combined eye-head tracking is relatively spared [2]. Unilateral lesions can cause ipsilateral deficits in smooth pursuit and gaze holding [3].

In humans, the paraflocculus has a major role in smooth pursuit, while the flocculus is more involved in the control of vestibulo-ocular reflex (VOR). The patients with flocculus and paraflocculus lesions have impaired smooth pursuit (primarily manifest as decreased gain during steady tracking state) and VOR cancellation. Moreover, gaze-holding is also impaired because flocculus and paraflocculus provide constant feedbacks to the brainstem neural integrators, which normally optimize the gaze-holding function.

Lesions of flocculus and paraflocculus can also cause downbeat nystagmus (Fig. 7.1). It is believed there is physiological upward-downward asymmetry of the signal driving vertical pursuit; this asymmetry in the signal is to compensate for the downward bias driven by the gravity [4]. Moreover, the flocculus and para-flocculus Purkinje cells inhibit the vestibular nuclei that receive input from the anterior semicircular canals [5–8]. Loss of Purkinje inhibition to the vestibular neurons sets free the anterior semicircular canal input, thus the eyes drift upward followed by a corrective downward saccades leading to downbeat nystagmus. Another type of nystagmus could be seen is rebound nystagmus. It occurs after the eyes return to the center position from the eccentric gaze. In rebound nystagmus the fast phase is in the direction opposite to where the eyes returned. For example, when the eyes return from right gaze, the direction of fast phase in the rebound nystagmus will be towards left [9].

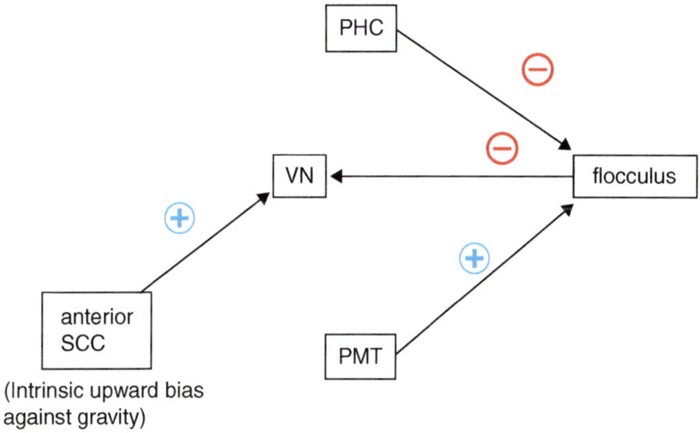

Fig. 7.1 Simplified illustration of the floccular pathways. Anterior semicircular canal (anterior SCC) has intrinsic upward bias signal which to make up for gravity pull. The flocculus is the integrator receiving signals from the perihypoglossal complex (PHC) and the paramedian tract cell groups (PMT). The flocculus normally inhibits vestibular nucleus (VN) to balance the intrinsic upward bias signal from anterior SCC

The flocculus and paraflocculus do not have a direct role in the generation of VOR. However, due to their tonic inhibition on the vestibular nuclei, the lesions of the flocculus and paraflocculus can disinhibit the anterior semicircular canal inputs affecting the VOR matrix [1, 10]. Different from the animal studies, active combined eye-head tracking are also impaired in patients with flocculus and paraflocculus lesion [11–13].

Clinically isolated flocculus and paraflocculus deficits can be explained by a strategic infarct involving the anterior inferior cerebellar artery (AICA) territory. However isolated involvement of the flocculus and paraflocculus, while sparing other regions supplied by AICA such as the dorsolateral pons and ipsilateral labyrinth is extremely rare. Literature reported in such patient population the eye exams demonstrated ipsilesional spontaneous nystagmus, which obeys Alexander's law and increases without visual fixation, clockwise torsional nystagmus (the top pole of the eyes beating towards right), contraversive ocular tilt reaction (might be acutely or later on), decreased VOR gain to contralesional rotations but normal caloric testing, impaired ipsiversive pursuit and VOR cancellation [14, 15]. Isolated flocculus syndrome was also described in critically ill patients due to herpes simplex virus type 1 (HSV1) encephalitis. The downbeat nystagmus was present, and was robust in primary gaze but attenuated during upgaze, suggestive of the flocculus involvement. In one of the two patients, FLAIR and T2-sequences of the brain MRI revealed cerebral lesions typical of HSV1, but also patchy hyperintensities in bilateral flocculi. Cerebrospinal fluid polymerase chain reaction confirmed HSV1 infection in one patient, and the encephalopathy and downbeat nystagmus gradually improved with acyclovir therapy.

Lesions of Nodulus and Ventral Uvula

The precision and accuracy of the VOR is fundamental for steady vision during locomotion. In addition to precise calibration of brainstem and semicircular canal function, the cerebellum is also critical for modulating the VOR matrix. The nodulus and ventral uvula are known to enhance the fidelity of VOR at low frequency rotations by implementing the concept called the velocity storage [16–19]. The velocity storage mechanism is dependent upon the GABA-B mediated inhibitory projections from the nodulus and ventral uvula [20, 21]. In humans the velocity storage is prominent for horizontal semicircular canal-driven rotations, but is relatively weak for the vertical canals [22]. One of the key functional implications of the velocity storage and its modulation by nodulus and ventral uvula is that such mechanism determines the body's internal estimate of gravity, a fundamental process to determine the direction of the VOR [23–26]. Acute deficits in nodulus and ventral uvula can be present in those with cerebellar strokes. In these patients the primary deficit can be gravity dependent nystagmus, where the direction of the nystagmus changes with the orientation of the head with respect to the gravity [27]. Selective nodulus and ventral uvula lesions can also lead to isolated downbeat nystagmus, latter can be due to the impaired modulation of the otolith-driven translational VOR [28, 29]. To differentiate the mechanism of downbeat nystagmus, whether it is due to the rotational VOR system (i.e. disinhibition of the anterior semicircular canal) or the translational VOR system, is to examine the eyes during eccentric horizontal gaze. During eccentric gaze, the presence of torsional nystagmus suggests semicircular canal origin; when such torsional nystagmus is absent then the likely the etiology is the nodulus-driven translational VOR system. Alternating skew deviation with elevation of the abducting eye or paroxysmal alternating skew deviation, tilt of the subjective visual vertical away from the side of the lesion, head-shaking-induced nystagmus (either direction changing or vertical) or position dependent horizontal nystagmus can all suggest acute lesion of nodulus and ventral uvula [30–35]. The acute lesions affecting the nodulus and ventral uvula can also manifest as isolated vertigo that can sometimes be position dependent. The proposed hypothesis depicted anatomically discrete but mechanistically identical velocity storage for the perception of angular motion. Isolated involvement of such perceptual pathways can cause acute onset of vertigo. In a cohort of critically ill patients with focal cerebellar lesions that only manifest as vertigo with absence of spontaneous nystagmus, the MRI revealed an area of acute infarct consistently involving dorsal aspect of the nodulus and ventral uvula [36]. When the infarct extended to the entire nodulus and ventral uvula, patients started to develop nystagmus with position dependence [36]. Periodic alternating nystagmus (PAN) is characterized by spontaneous horizontal nystagmus presenting in the primary gaze, and characteristically reverses its direction approximately every 2 min [37]. Such deficits are considered typical manifestation of the nodulus lesion and are responsive to the treatment with GABA-B agonist – baclofen [20, 24, 38].

Lesions of the Dorsal Vermis and Fastigial nuclei (FOR, Fastigial Oculomotor Region)

The dorsal vermis and FOR have a key role in modulating the matrix of saccades (Fig. 7.2). The Fig. 7.2 demonstrated how dorsal vermis and fastigial nucleus work together to modulate saccades matrix. Experimental lesions either dorsal vermis or the fastigial nuclei result in saccadic dysmetria. Bilaterally symmetric lesion of vermis causes hypometria; and lesions affecting the fastigial nuclei cause hypermetria [39–43]. Although such deficits frequently affect the horizontal saccades, prominent vertical saccadic dysmetria are present [44]. Although isolated fastigial lesion is extremely rare clinically, the Wallenberg syndrome is a functional mimic of ipsilateral fastigial lesion. In Wallenberg syndrome, as described at length in the chapter on medulla, lesion of

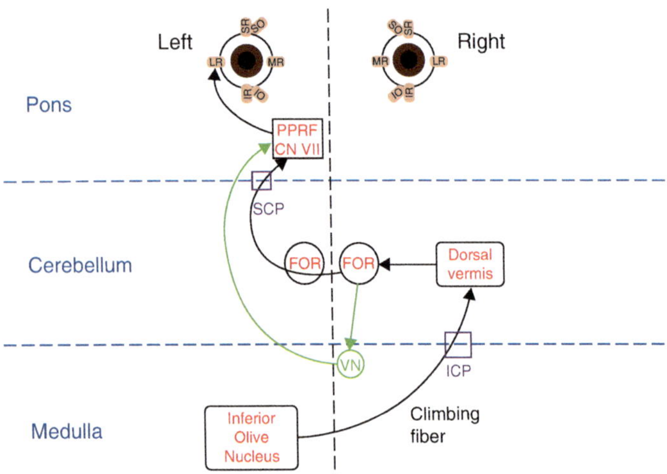

Fig. 7.2 Schematic outline of the pathways connecting dorsal vermis and fastigial nuclei (FOR) with other eye movement structures. Inferior olive nucleus sends inhibitory axons to the dorsal vermis via climbing fibers passing through inferior cerebellar peduncle (ICP). Dorsal vermis inhibits the FOR. Latter acts as an initializer and a brake for saccades matrix

inferior cerebellar peduncle leads to disinhibition of the dorsal vermis resulting in the inhibition of the fastigial nucleus.

Dorsal vermis lesions commonly leads to dysmetria of the saccades made to externally triggered visual targets, but they are not seen in internally generated saccades (in the absence of a visual target) such as during scanning of a visual scene [45, 46]. Lesions of dorsal vermis and the fastigial nucleus also affect the ability to initiate smooth pursuit eye movement (i.e. the acceleration) [47, 48]. In dorsal vermis lesion, the pursuit deficits are ipsilateral. In addition to abnormal initiation, the pursuit velocity is also impaired [49, 50]. Unlike dorsal vermis, the fastigial lesion impairs the acceleration of the contralateral pursuits [51]. Clinically, fastigial lesions are generally bilateral because of their proximity and axon crossing. Therefore it is possible to have marked saccadic hypermetria but minimally impaired smooth pursuit because each of the bilateral fastigial nuclei causes opposing effects on the pursuit hence bilateral lesions "cancel" the deficits [45, 52].

Summary

In this chapter, we reviewed the critical role of cerebellum in eye movements. Functionally, cerebellum can be divided into three regions and therefore three groups of syndromes have been proposed based on this division: the syndrome of flocculus and paraflocculus, the syndrome of nodulus and ventral uvula and the syndrome of dorsal vermis and fastigial nuclei. Despite theoretical segregation, there is a significant overlap within clinical manifestation because a disease process is usually not confined to one critical area. To simplify, we will recap the common presentations of each syndrome. Lesions involving flocculus and paraflocculus lead to abnormal smooth pursuit, vestibular ocular reflex and downbeat nystagmus. Lesions of nodulus and ventral uvula characteristically lead to periodic alternating nystagmus because they are known as the velocity storage mechanism. They might also cause downbeat nystagmus. The syndrome of dorsal vermis and fastigial nuclei manifest as dysmetric saccades.

References

1. Zee DS, Yamazaki A, Butler PH, Gucer G. Effects of ablation of flocculus and paraflocculus of eye movements in primate. J Neurophysiol. 1981;46(4):878–99.
2. Belton T, McCrea RA. Role of the cerebellar flocculus region in the coordination of eye and head movements during gaze pursuit. J Neurophysiol. 2000;84(3):1614–26.
3. Straube A, Scheuerer W, Eggert T. Unilateral cerebellar lesions affect initiation of ipsilateral smooth pursuit eye movements in humans. Ann Neurol. 1997;42(6):891–8.
4. Pierrot-Deseilligny C, Milea D. Vertical nystagmus: clinical facts and hypotheses. Brain. 2005;128(Pt 6):1237–46.
5. Marti S, Straumann D, Glasauer S. The origin of downbeat nystagmus: an asymmetry in the distribution of on-directions of vertical gaze-velocity Purkinje cells. Ann N Y Acad Sci. 2005;1039:548–53.
6. Kalla R, Deutschlander A, Hufner K, Stephan T, Jahn K, Glasauer S, et al. Detection of floccular hypometabolism in downbeat nystagmus by fMRI. Neurology. 2006;66(2):281–3.
7. Hufner K, Stephan T, Kalla R, Deutschlander A, Wagner J, Holtmannspotter M, et al. Structural and functional MRIs disclose cerebellar pathologies in idiopathic downbeat nystagmus. Neurology. 2007;69(11):1128–35.
8. Fukushima K, Kaneko CR. Vestibular integrators in the oculomotor system. Neurosci Res. 1995;22(3):249–58.
9. Kheradmand A, Zee DS. Cerebellum and ocular motor control. Front Neurol. 2011;2:53.
10. Takemori S, Cohen B. Loss of visual suppression of vestibular nystagmus after flocculus lesions. Brain Res. 1974;72(2):213–24.
11. Waterston JA, Barnes GR, Grealy MA. A quantitative study of eye and head movements during smooth pursuit in patients with cerebellar disease. Brain. 1992;115(Pt 5):1343–58.
12. Buttner U, Grundei T. Gaze-evoked nystagmus and smooth pursuit deficits: their relationship studied in 52 patients. J Neurol. 1995;242(6):384–9.
13. Grant MP, Leigh RJ, Seidman SH, Riley DE, Hanna JP. Comparison of predictable smooth ocular and combined eye-head tracking behaviour in patients with lesions affecting the brainstem and cerebellum. Brain. 1992;115(Pt 5):1323–42.
14. Park HK, Kim JS, Strupp M, Zee DS. Isolated floccular infarction: impaired vestibular responses to horizontal head impulse. J Neurol. 2013;260(6):1576–82.
15. Yacovino DA, Akly MP, Luis L, Zee DS. The floccular syndrome: dynamic changes in eye movements and vestibulo-ocular reflex in isolated infarction of the cerebellar flocculus. Cerebellum. 2018;17(2):122–31.

16. Cohen B, Helwig D, Raphan T. Baclofen and velocity storage: a model of the effects of the drug on the vestibulo-ocular reflex in the rhesus monkey. J Physiol. 1987;393:703–25.
17. Solomon D, Cohen B. Stimulation of the nodulus and uvula discharges velocity storage in the vestibulo-ocular reflex. Exp Brain Res. 1994;102(1):57–68.
18. Walker MF, Tian J, Shan X, Tamargo RJ, Ying H, Zee DS. The cerebellar nodulus/uvula integrates otolith signals for the translational vestibulo-ocular reflex. PLoS One. 2010;5(11):e13981.
19. Beh SC, Frohman TC, Frohman EM. Cerebellar control of eye movements. J Neuroophthalmol. 2017;37(1):87–98.
20. Dai M, Raphan T, Cohen B. Effects of baclofen on the angular vestibulo-ocular reflex. Exp Brain Res. 2006;171(2):262–71.
21. Shaikh AG, Marti S, Tarnutzer AA, Palla A, Crawford TO, Zee DS, et al. Effects of 4-aminopyridine on nystagmus and vestibulo-ocular reflex in ataxia-telangiectasia. J Neurol. 2013;260(11):2728–35.
22. Shaikh AG, Palla A, Marti S, Olasagasti I, Optican LM, Zee DS, et al. Role of cerebellum in motion perception and vestibulo-ocular reflex-similarities and disparities. Cerebellum. 2013;12(1):97–107.
23. Angelaki DE, Shaikh AG, Green AM, Dickman JD. Neurons compute internal models of the physical laws of motion. Nature. 2004;430(6999):560–4.
24. Shaikh AG, Meng H, Angelaki DE. Multiple reference frames for motion in the primate cerebellum. J Neurosci. 2004;24(19):4491–7.
25. Shaikh AG, Ghasia FF, Dickman JD, Angelaki DE. Properties of cerebellar fastigial neurons during translation, rotation, and eye movements. J Neurophysiol. 2005;93(2):853–63.
26. Shaikh AG, Marti S, Tarnutzer AA, Palla A, Crawford TO, Straumann D, et al. Ataxia telangiectasia: a "disease model" to understand the cerebellar control of vestibular reflexes. J Neurophysiol. 2011;105(6):3034–41.
27. Shaikh AG, Miller BR, Sundararajan S, Katirji B. Gravity-dependent nystagmus and inner-ear dysfunction suggest anterior and posterior inferior cerebellar artery infarct. J Stroke Cerebrovasc Dis. 2014;23(4):788–90.
28. Patel VR, Zee DS. The cerebellum in eye movement control: nystagmus, coordinate frames and disconjugacy. Eye (Lond). 2015;29(2):191–5.
29. Marti S, Palla A, Straumann D. Gravity dependence of ocular drift in patients with cerebellar downbeat nystagmus. Ann Neurol. 2002;52(6):712–21.
30. Radtke A, Bronstein AM, Gresty MA, Faldon M, Taylor W, Stevens JM, et al. Paroxysmal alternating skew deviation and nystagmus after partial destruction of the uvula. J Neurol Neurosurg Psychiatry. 2001;70(6):790–3.
31. Tsuda H, Nagamata M, Tanaka K. Alternating skew deviation due to hemorrhage in the cerebellar vermis. Intern Med. 2012;51(19):2793–6.

32. Tarnutzer AA, Wichmann W, Straumann D, Bockisch CJ. The cerebellar nodulus: perceptual and ocular processing of graviceptive input. Ann Neurol. 2015;77(2):343–7.
33. Kim HA, Lee H, Yi HA, Lee SR, Lee SY, Baloh RW. Pattern of otolith dysfunction in posterior inferior cerebellar artery territory cerebellar infarction. J Neurol Sci. 2009;280(1–2):65–70.
34. Kim HA, Yi HA, Lee H. Apogeotropic central positional nystagmus as a sole sign of nodular infarction. Neurol Sci. 2012;33(5):1189–91.
35. Lee HJ, Kim ES, Kim M, Chu H, Ma HI, Lee JS, et al. Isolated horizontal positional nystagmus from a posterior fossa lesion. Ann Neurol. 2014;76(6):905–10.
36. Shaikh AG. Motion perception without Nystagmus–a novel manifestation of cerebellar stroke. J Stroke Cerebrovasc Dis. 2014;23(5):1148–56.
37. Leigh RJ, Robinson DA, Zee DS. A hypothetical explanation for periodic alternating nystagmus: instability in the optokinetic-vestibular system. Ann N Y Acad Sci. 1981;374:619–35.
38. Waespe W, Cohen B, Raphan T. Dynamic modification of the vestibulo-ocular reflex by the nodulus and uvula. Science. 1985;228(4696):199–202.
39. Robinson FR, Straube A, Fuchs AF. Role of the caudal fastigial nucleus in saccade generation. II. Effects of muscimol inactivation. J Neurophysiol. 1993;70(5):1741–58.
40. Takagi M, Zee DS, Tamargo RJ. Effects of lesions of the oculomotor vermis on eye movements in primate: saccades. J Neurophysiol. 1998;80(4):1911–31.
41. Kojima Y, Soetedjo R, Fuchs AF. Effect of inactivation and disinhibition of the oculomotor vermis on saccade adaptation. Brain Res. 2011;1401:30–9.
42. Straube A, Scheuerer W, Robinson FR, Eggert T. Temporary lesions of the caudal deep cerebellar nucleus in nonhuman primates. Gain, offset, and ocular alignment. Ann N Y Acad Sci. 2009;1164:119–26.
43. Selhorst JB, Stark L, Ochs AL, Hoyt WF. Disorders in cerebellar ocular motor control. I. Saccadic overshoot dysmetria. An oculographic, control system and clinico-anatomical analysis. Brain. 1976;99(3):497–508.
44. Serrano-Munuera C, Corral-Juan M, Stevanin G, San Nicolas H, Roig C, Corral J, et al. New subtype of spinocerebellar ataxia with altered vertical eye movements mapping to chromosome 1p32. JAMA Neurol. 2013;70(6):764–71.
45. Büttner U, Straube A. The effect of cerebellar midline lesions on eye movements. Neuro-Ophthalmology. 1995;15(2):75–82.
46. Straube A, Deubel H, Spuler A, Büttner U. Differential effect of a bilateral deep cerebellar nuclei lesion on externally and internally triggered saccades in humans. Neuro-Ophthalmology. 1995;15(2):67–74.

47. Takagi M, Zee DS, Tamargo RJ. Effects of lesions of the oculomotor cerebellar vermis on eye movements in primate: smooth pursuit. J Neurophysiol. 2000;83(4):2047–62.
48. Dash S, Catz N, Dicke PW, Thier P. Encoding of smooth-pursuit eye movement initiation by a population of vermal Purkinje cells. Cereb Cortex. 2012;22(4):877–91.
49. Vahedi K, Rivaud S, Amarenco P, Pierrot-Deseilligny C. Horizontal eye movement disorders after posterior vermis infarctions. J Neurol Neurosurg Psychiatry. 1995;58(1):91–4.
50. Nawrot M, Rizzo M. Motion perception deficits from midline cerebellar lesions in human. Vis Res. 1995;35(5):723–31.
51. Robinson FR, Straube A, Fuchs AF. Participation of caudal fastigial nucleus in smooth pursuit eye movements. II. Effects of muscimol inactivation. J Neurophysiol. 1997;78(2):848–59.
52. Moschner C, Zangemeister WH, Demer JL. Anticipatory smooth eye movements of high velocity triggered by large target steps: normal performance and effect of cerebellar degeneration. Vis Res. 1996;36(9):1341–8.

Eye Movements and Vestibular Dysfunction: Lesions of Pons

8

Important anatomical structures in the pons participating in the control of eye movements include the abducens nucleus, paramedian pontine reticular formation (PPRF), medial longitudinal fasciculus (MLF), and the rostral portion of the vestibular nucleus. The compact organization of the pons makes it amenable to get significant clinical deficit despite small lesions such as lacunar infarcts. Medical manifestations of critical illness, such as malignant hypertension, can also result in pontine dysfunction. Lesions affecting each pontine nuclei themselves can cause specific clinical presentation; but sometimes (larger deficits) present with constellation of symptoms leading to specific syndromic entities. This chapter outlines the range of ocular motor deficits that are expected from the lesions affecting the pontine nuclei (Table 8.1).

Abducens Palsy

The abducens nerve (cranial nerve VI) innervates the lateral rectus muscle of the eye. The abducens palsy leads to ipsilateral abduction deficit. Simplistically considered the sole abductor, the lateral rectus also has small vertical control. As a result the abducens palsy may present with small vertical deviations, typically the hypermetria during saccades on the side ipsilateral to the lesion [1, 2] (Fig. 8.1). The Fig. 8.1 depicts the cross section of the pons.

A. Shaikh, F. Wang, *Eye Movements in the Critical Care Setting*,
https://doi.org/10.1007/978-3-030-70221-2_8

Table 8.1 Ocular motor dysfunction in pontine lesions

Abducens nucleus	Conjugate ipsilateral horizontal gaze palsy Horizontal gaze-evoked nystagmus when looking contralaterally Contralateral gaze deviation in acute phase Slow ipsilateral saccades
Abducens nerve fascicle	Esotropia of ipsilateral eye and inability of ipsilateral eye abduction
PPRF	Horizontal saccades palsy towards the lesion side Horizontal gaze-evoked nystagmus when looking contralaterally Contralateral gaze deviation in acute phase
MLF	Internuclear ophthalmoplegia (INO) (weakness or paralysis of adduction on the side of MLF lesion during conjugate movements) Dissociated horizontal "nystagmus" of abducting eye contralateral to the MLF lesion Preserved convergence Ocular tilt reaction (ipsilateral hyper-deviation) Dissociated vertical-torsional nystagmus

The abducens nucleus is in the dorsal medial aspect of the pons and its nerve fascicles travel ventrally and exit at the level of pontomedullary junction. The abducens nucleus has two types of neurons, the motoneurons innervating the ipsilateral lateral rectus, and the interneurons that join the medial longitudinal fasciculus (MLF). Lesions affecting the abducens nerve fascicle cause ipsilateral lateral rectus palsy, leading to disconjugate eye movement. In contrast, the abducens nucleus injury involves both the motoneurons and the interneurons, leading to impairment in horizontal conjugate gaze deviation [3–9]. In cases of abducens nuclear or nerve palsy, the vertical eye movements and convergence are relatively spared. The saccades, pursuits, optokinetic and vestibular movements are also preserved in the contralateral hemifield, but they are affected in the direction towards the lesion side. These deficits are due to the fact that all eye movements follow final common pathway, and the abducens nucleus has a critical role in it (Fig. 8.2). Figure 8.2 demonstrates the simplified organization of the saccade pathway. For example, in the case of a lesion

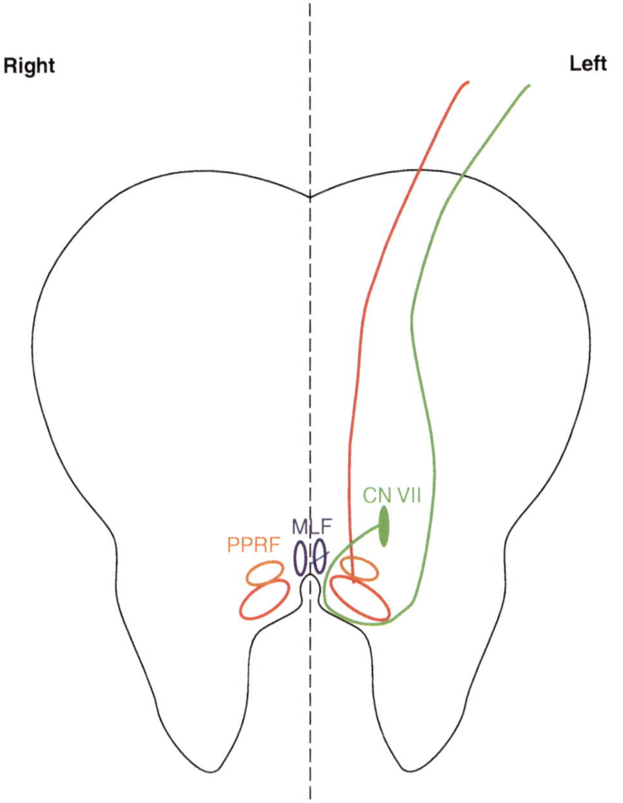

Fig. 8.1 The schematic demonstration of the cross section of the pons. Abducens nucleus is in the proximity of the midline with PPRF in its adjacency. The abducens nerve fascicles travels ventrally and leaves at pontomedullary junction. The facial nerve initially travels medially and dorsally, then loops around the abducens nucleus and travels ventrally and laterally, then exits at the pontomedullary junction

affecting the left abducens nucleus, the saccades from center to the left are obviously affected. The saccades from the center to right are preserved, because they depend on the projections from the excitatory burst neurons (EBN) of the right paramedian pontine reticular formation (PPRF) to the intact right abducens

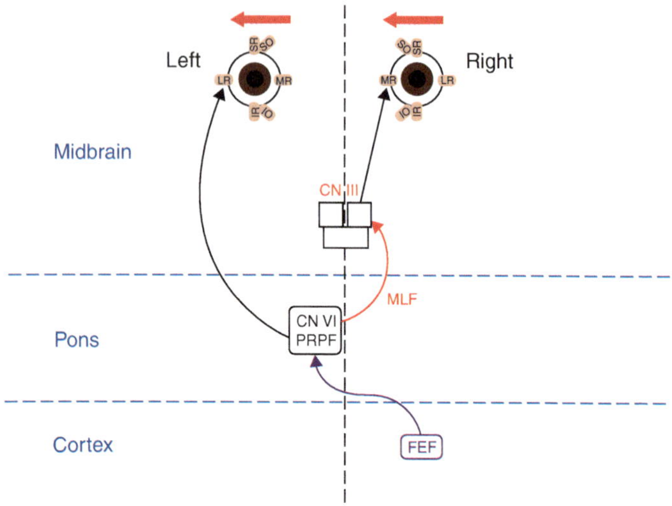

Fig. 8.2 The diagram depicts the connection between the frontal eye filed (FEF) and end saccadic pathway. Right FEF activates the left abducens nucleus (CN VI) and paramedian pontine reticular formation (PPRF) which then activates right lateral rectus (LR) and left medial rectus (MR) via medial longitudinal fasciculus (MLF). In the end both eyes make saccadic movements towards right side

nucleus and subsequently to the left oculomotor nucleus. The saccades from the right gaze to center are slow because they are accomplished by abrupt relaxation of the antagonist muscles (right lateral rectus and left medial rectus) due to projections from the inhibitory burst neurons (IBN) of the left medullary reticular formation to the intact, right abducens nucleus. Thus, eyes returning to the center from right gaze is a function of antagonist muscle relaxation rather than agonist contraction. Contralateral gaze shift can be present with horizontal gaze-evoked nystagmus, likely secondary to the interruption of fibers passing through the medial vestibular nucleus providing the eye position signal to the contralateral abducens nucleus or due to the lesions of the fibers from the paramedian tract (PMT) cell groups [4]. Lesions restricted to the abducens nucleus are rare. The facial nerve fascicle loop around the abducens nucleus before exiting at pontomedullary junction, therefore it is not uncommon to find ipsilateral lower motor neuron facial palsy in addition to abducens nerve palsy (Fig. 8.1) [10, 11].

Lesions of Paramedian Pontine Reticular Formation (PPRF)

The PPRF mainly consists of four groups of neuron axons, excitatory burst neurons (EBN), inhibitory burst neurons (IBN), long-lead burst neurons (LLBN) and omnipause neurons [12]. The most common presentation of the PPRF lesion is slowing of ipsilateral horizontal saccades [13]. The extent of PPRF lesion determines the severity or slowness of saccades. The saccade velocity is determined by the interactions of IBN, EBN, and the omnipause neurons. Selective lesion primarily affecting the EBNs cause saccadic slowing, but if the lesion also extends to caudal region involving the IBNs then the saccades get even slower or absent [4, 14]. Vertical saccades can be slow and misdirected obliquely away from the lesion side due to imbalanced horizontal components [15].

Smooth pursuit and slow phase of optokinetic nystagmus are usually preserved due to different end motor pathways in the brainstem. Nevertheless, it was reported that more rostral pontine lesions tend to cause ipsilateral smooth pursuit deficits, whereas caudal pontine lesions cause contralateral deficits [16, 17]. It was also suggested that basal lesions in the pons can affect ipsilateral or bilateral pursuit due to involvement of pontine nuclei [18–21].

Bilateral PPRF lesions are rare, however they were described in the syndrome of selective saccade palsy following cardiac surgery, especially aortic valve replacement and after the dissection of the thoracic aorta. This cardiogenic syndrome, characterized by selective saccade palsy, spares other forms of eye movements and it can be seen in those who are admitted to critical care units [22–28]. In patients with cardiogenic saccade palsy have slowing in all directions, and it affects voluntary saccades as well as reflexive (i.e., the quick phase of nystagmus). The extreme cases have the complete loss of saccades. In responding to optokinetic stimuli, the patients could make smooth tracking movement to the far eccentric gaze without the ability to generate fast phases to bring the eyes back to center. Blinking and head thrusts can aid the range and speed of voluntary saccades in some patients, but most affected patients remain permanently visually disabled by loss of their ability to shift their direction of gaze voluntarily. The pathophysiology of this syndrome is still under further investigation, however it was postulated to be secondary to hypoperfusion to the paramedian pons. Consistent with this hypothesis, autopsy showed the evidence of neuronal loss and gliosis confined to the regions of the omnipause neurons and excitatory burst neurons; other parts of pons were spared. In animal experiments, perineuronal nets made of chondroitin sulfate proteoglycans surrounding saccadic burst neurons and omnipause neurons were discovered [29]. These structures are extremely vulnerable to hypoperfusion [30, 31].

Omnipause neurons, located in the nucleus raphe interpositus in the paramedian structure of pons, also project to the vertical burst neurons via medial longitudinal fasciculus [32]. As a consequence the bilateral pontine lesions can also impair vertical eye movements, especially the vertical saccades [22, 33–37]. In otherwords midline pontine lesions involving the omnipause neurons can cause omnidirectional saccadic slowing.

Medial Longitudinal Fasciculus (MLF)

Medial longitudinal fasciculus houses axons for horizontal, vertical and torsional eye movements. For horizontal gaze, the axons carry signals from the abducens interneurons projecting to contralateral medial rectus motoneurons in the oculomotor nucleus (Fig. 8.2). Whereas for vertical and torsional gaze, axons from vestibular nuclei carry smooth pursuit, rotational and linear vestibulo-ocular reflex (VOR) and steady gaze holding signal projecting to oculomotor, trochlear nuclei, interstitial nucleus of Cajal and rostral interstitial nucleus of MLF (riMLF).

MLF lesions, commonly caused by infarction and demyelination, present with characteristic neuro-ophthalmologic manifestation, the internuclear ophthalmoplegia (INO). The most important sign of INO is reduced or absent adduction of ipsilateral eye. When naming the laterality of INO, the side of MLF lesion is the same as the eye that is unable to adduct. In some minor lesions, there might only be slowed adduction saccades, called "adduction lag". Therefore, making a clinical diagnosis of INO relies on examining saccades between two distant targets and paying attention to speed of the adduction velocity, or by using hand-held optokinetic drum or tape [38]. When INO is caused by demyelination, the affected nerve fiber is unable to transmit high-frequency signal for saccades but can still be able to sustain low-frequency discharges for other slower types of eye movements. Such result is reflected as pulse-step mismatch dissociation, the saccade speed is reduced out of proportion to the range of adduction. In addition to adduction paresis, there can be abnormalities of abduction saccades in the affected eye, particularly hypometria with the centripetal drifts [39] and slowing [40].

The other core symptom is abduction nystagmus of the contralateral eye [41]. So far there are two plausible hypotheses. One is the adaptation mechanism. The brain attempts to compensate for the adduction weakness. As a result there is an increased commensurate amount of innervation to the adducting eye. According to the Hering's law of equal innervation, the compensatory innervation must be accompanied by addition of equal amount of innervation to the normal abducting eye. Thus, the end result leads to overshoot saccades and backward, post-saccadic drift of the abducting eye, the abduction nystagmus [42, 43]. In this case, the oscillation is initiated by saccades hence it is not a true nystagmus. The post-saccadic drift should be brief and small, and the waveform should be independent of how far eccentric the abduction eye is. The other probable mechanism is dissociated gaze-evoked nystagmus which is more prevalent in the abducting eye due to adduction weakness. This is a "true" nystagmus, it is relatively persistent, and the post-saccadic drift has the intention to bring the eye back to the center if it is not interrupted by corrective saccades. The dissociated nystagmus is putatively generated by lesions involving the fibers near the MLF carrying information from floccular complexes [44].

The INO is frequently associated with skew deviation, or ocular tilt reaction. Typically, the higher eye is on the side of MLF lesion [45, 46]. This is due to disruption of the graviceptive pathway carrying information from the contralateral vestibular system ascending in the MLF. The associated adduction defect and intorsion of the higher eye is often distinguishable from the trochlear nerve palsy where the higher eye is extorted.

Dissociated torsional-vertical nystagmus can also be present in the MLF lesion. There might be three types of vertical components. The most common form is upbeat in both eyes but greater in the contralesional eye. Following is the seesaw nystagmus characterized by the downbeat in the higher eye on the lesion side and upbeat in the lower eye on the opposite side. The least common type is downbeat in both eyes but greater in the higher eye on the lesion side. Three speculations were proposed for these observations. First, posterior semicircular canal projections are confined to the MLF whereas anterior semicircular canal has extra-MLF pathways. Second, involvement of utriculo-ocular pathways also contributes to ocular tilt reaction. Third, there is concurrent lesion involving the nerve fibers of paramedian tracts that carry the information related to the vertical gaze holding [47–49]. The VOR in INO can be asymmetric with rapid head rotations [50–52]. Bilateral INO often causes additional findings such as gaze-evoked vertical nystagmus, impaired vertical pursuit, and decreased vertical vestibular responses [53–55].

Defect of vergence in patients with INO are variable; so far there was no single universally accepted explanation. When convergence is intact in the setting of absent adduction with conjugate eye movements, a more caudal lesion with preservation of medial rectus motoneurons has been assumed. The convergence is affected in rostral lesions due to the involvement of oculomotor nucleus or pretectal structures [56].

Bilateral INO or wall-eyed bilateral INO (WEBINO) presents with bilateral exotropia [53]. In addition to aforementioned abnormalities related to MLF, vertical optokinetic nystagmus vertical smooth pursuit is also impaired. VOR cancellation might also be impaired when there is some sparing of the vertical VOR. Vertical gaze holding is also impaired, probably because of involvement of the projections between the vestibular nuclei and the interstitial nucleus of Cajal, and the paramedian tracts.

One-and-Half Syndrome and Its Variants

Lesions involving the abducens nucleus with or without PPRF and adjacent MLF crossed from contralateral abducens nucleus on one side of brain cause an ipsilateral horizontal gaze palsy and INO, thus the only motion preserved is the abduction of the contralateral eye, i.e. one-and-half syndrome (Fig. 8.3) [57]. The Fig. 8.3 depicted right-sided one and half syndrome. Some patients may have an exotropia of contralateral eye at primary gaze due to paralytic pontine exotropia [58–60]. Dissociated abducting nystagmus could still be observed in the contralateral eye. Occasionally, ipsilateral horizontal vestibular responses may be preserved, even though patients are unable to perform voluntary horizontal eye movements [61]. This indicates that the lesion

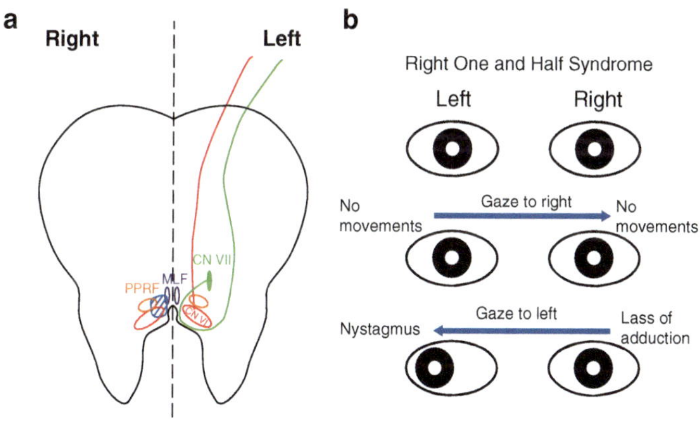

Fig. 8.3 Schematic of right one-and-half syndrome. (**a**) Lesion involves medial longitudinal fasciculus (MLF), abducens nucleus (CN VI) and or paramedian pontine reticular formation (PPRF) on the right side. (**b**) Eye movement abnormalities in right one and half syndrome

is likely located either in the more rostral part or the very caudal part of PPRF, with preservation of the projections from vestibular nucleus to abducens nucleus [61, 62]. Again, even in the one-and-half syndrome, vergence can be spared. Rarely ocular bobbing is seen in one and half syndrome [63]. Presence of peripheral facial nerve palsy on the same side of one-and-half syndrome advices the involvement of abducens nucleus, genu of facial nerve fascicle and adjacent MLF, thus it has been called eight-and-half syndrome [64–66]. Fifteen-and-half syndrome is when bilateral facial nerve palsy appears in association with one-and-half syndrome [67]. Rarely supranuclear facial nerve palsy is also seen when some patients have corticobulbar tract branching off below the level of pontomedullary junction and loop upwards through pontine tegmentum to reach the caudal half of facial nucleus on the contralateral side [68]. Added involvement of ipsilateral cochlear nucleus with facial nerve leads to "sixteen-and-half syndrome" [69, 70]. Bilateral facial nerve palsy and one-and-half syndrome, plus ipsilateral fifth nerve palsy leads to twenty-and-half syndrome [71]. When there is an involvement of bilateral eighth nerve, ipsilateral seventh nerve and one-and-half syndrome, it becomes twenty-four-and-half syndrome [72].

Pontine Stroke Syndromes

Amongst many pontine stroke syndromes, only a few affect the eye movements. These ocular motor pontine syndromes are discussed below (Table 8.2).

Raymond Syndrome

The Raymond syndrome is characterized as ipsilateral fascicular sixth nerve palsy and contralateral hemiparesis or hemiplegia due to the involvement of pyramidal tracts (Fig. 8.4) [73–75]. The Raymond syndrome typically affects the caudal ventral pons. Involvement of corticobulbar tract cause contralateral central facial droop [76].

Table 8.2 Pontine stroke syndromes with ocular motor abnormalities

Raymond Syndrome	Caudal ventral pons: Abducens nerve fascicle Corticospinal tract ±Corticobulbar tract	Ipsilateral eye abduction palsy Contralateral hemiparesis/ hemiplegia ±Contralateral central facial palsy
Millard-Gubler Syndrome	Caudal ventral pons: Abducens nerve fascicle Facial nerve fascicle Corticospinal tract	Ipsilateral eye abduction palsy Ipsilateral peripheral facial palsy Contralateral hemiparesis/ hemiplegia
Foville Syndrome	Caudal tegmental pons: Abducens nucleus PPRF Facial nerve fascicle Corticospinal tract	Ipsilateral conjugate gaze palsy Ipsilateral peripheral facial palsy Contralateral hemiparesis/ hemiplegia
Raymond-Cestan Syndrome	Rostral tegmental pons: Medial lemniscus MLF Cortical spinal tract Superior/middle cerebellar peduncle	Ipsilateral internuclear ophthalmoplegia (INO) Contralateral ataxia Contralateral hemiparesis/ hemiplegia

Millard-Gubler Syndrome

The Millard-Gubler syndrome is more extensive lesion of the caudal ventral pons involving sixth and seventh cranial nerve along with corticospinal tract (Fig. 8.5). The clinical manifestation includes ipsilateral sixth nerve palsy, peripheral facial palsy, and contralateral hemiparesis or hemiplegia [77, 78].

Foville Syndrome

The Fovielle syndrome is the caudal tegmental (dorsal) pontine lesion involving the abducens nucleus, PPRF, the seventh nerve fascicle and corticospinal tract (Fig. 8.6). The typical clinical

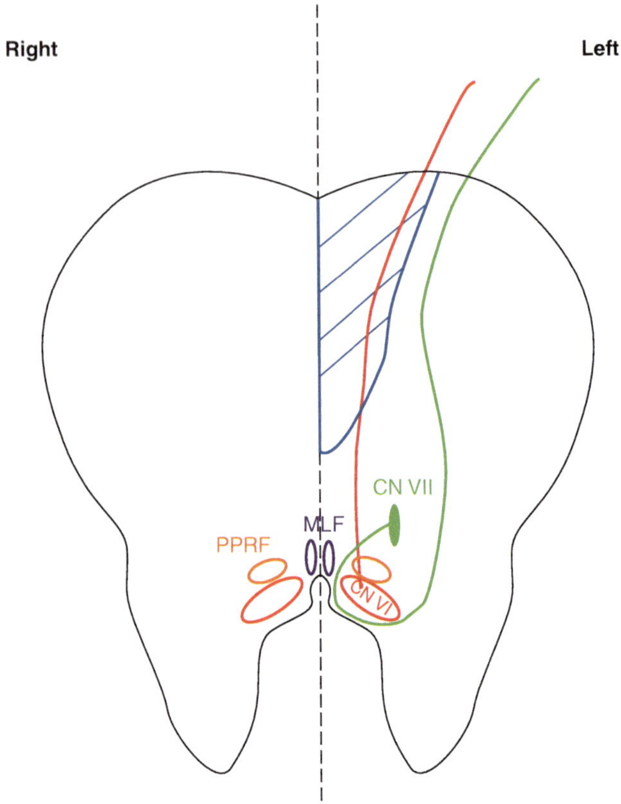

Fig. 8.4 Illustration of the Raymond Syndrome, with a lesion involving fascicle of abducens nerve (CN VI) as well as corticospinal tract ± corticobulbar tract

presentations include ipsilateral conjugate gaze palsy, peripheral facial palsy, and contralateral hemiparesis or hemiplegia [77].

Raymond-Cestan Syndrome

The Raymond-Cestan syndrome is a more extensive rostral lesion that also involves tegmental (dorsal) pons (Fig. 8.7). Involvement of corticospinal tract, medial lemniscus, medial longitudinal fas-

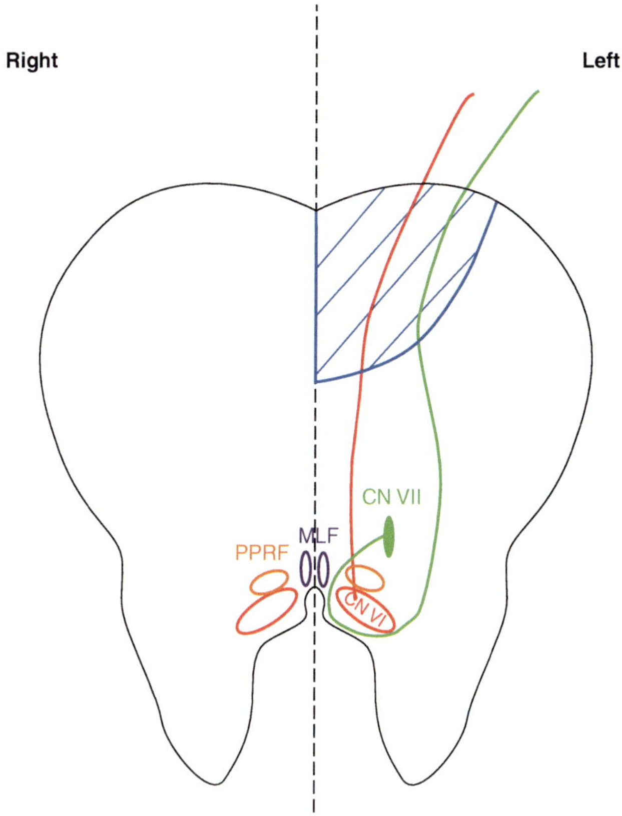

Fig. 8.5 Millard-Gubler Syndrome is diagrammatically illustrated. In this syndrome the more extensive ventral pontine lesion involves the fascicles of abducens (CN VI) and facial (CN VII) nerves, as well as corticospinal tract and corticobulbar tract

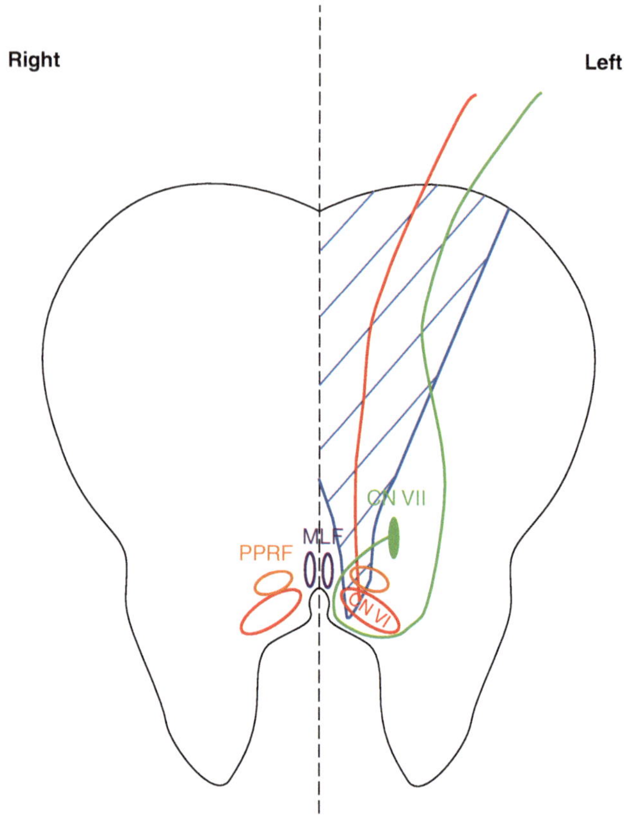

Fig. 8.6 Illustration of the Foville Syndrome where a pontine lesion extends from ventral to dorsal and involve abducens nucleus (CN VI) but spares the ipsilateral medial longitudinal fasciculus (MLF). Fascicle of facial nerve (CN VII), corticospinal and corticobulbar tracts are also involved in such extensive lesion

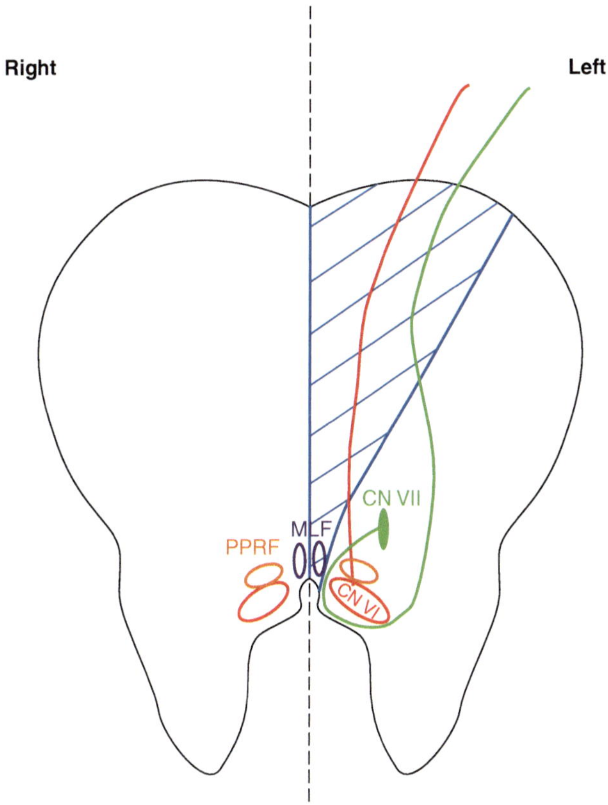

Fig. 8.7 The diagrammatic illustration of the Raymond-Cestan Syndrome. This type of extensive pontine lesion however with the involvement of medial longitudinal fasciculus (MLF) but spares abducens nucleus (CN VI)

ciculus, and superior/middle cerebellar peduncle gives rise to a constellation of symptoms including but not limited to ipsilateral INO, contralateral hemiparesis/hemiplegia and ataxia [77, 79].

Summary

In this chapter, we reviewed the critical role of pons with regards to eye movements. Important structures in the pons include abducens nucleus and its fascicle, paramedian pontine reticular formation (PPRF) and medial longitudinal fasciculus (MLF). They key difference to discern abducens nuclear palsy from nerve fascicle palsy is the involvement of contralateral eye. In abducens nerve fascicle lesion, only ipsilateral abduction is impaired. PPRF lesions can cause ipsiversive saccades palsy. One-and-half syndrome occurs when the lesion extends to the adjacent MLF. Internuclear ophthalmoplegia (INO) occurs if only the MLF is involved. We finally reviewed the common pontine stroke syndromes affecting the eye movements including Raymond syndrome, Millard-Gubler syndrome, Foville syndrome, and Raymond-Cestan syndrome.

References

1. Wong AM, Tweed D, Sharpe JA. Vertical misalignment in unilateral sixth nerve palsy. Ophthalmology. 2002;109(7):1315–25.
2. Pihlblad MS, Demer JL. Hypertropia in unilateral isolated abducens palsy. J AAPOS. 2014;18(3):235–40.
3. Saitou N, Takahashi J, Kashima Y, Ishikawa H. Horizontal gaze palsy due to lesion of the abducens nucleus detected with magnetic resonance imaging. Nippon Ganka Gakkai Zasshi. 1995;99(5):624–7.
4. Muri RM, Chermann JF, Cohen L, Rivaud S, Pierrot-Deseilligny C. Ocular motor consequences of damage to the abducens nucleus area in humans. J Neuroophthalmol. 1996;16(3):191–5.
5. Hirose G, Furui K, Yoshioka A, Sakai K. Unilateral conjugate gaze palsy due to a lesion of the abducens nucleus. Clinical and neuroradiological correlations. J Clin Neuroophthalmol. 1993;13(1):54–8.
6. Lhermitte F, Pages M. Abducens nucleus syndrome due to pontine haemorrhage. Cerebrovasc Dis. 2006;22(4):284–5.

7. Saiki M, Matsubara T, Suzuki K, Okamura M, Takekawa H, Nakamura T, et al. Conjugate eye deviation due to pontine infarction: report of 2 cases. eNeurologicalSci. 2018;11:1–2.
8. Hamasaki S, Motomura M, Koga H, Nakamura T, Yoshimura T. Persistent lateral gaze palsy and abducens nerve palsy due to pontine infarction. Rinsho Shinkeigaku. 1998;38(4):344–6.
9. Uemura J, Shibazaki K, Inoue T, Iguchi Y, Kimura K. A case of pontine infarction presenting with conjugate deviation and unilateral conjugate gaze palsy. Rinsho Shinkeigaku. 2007;47(5):231–3.
10. Roh JK, Kim BK, Chung JM. Combined peripheral facial and abducens nerve palsy caused by caudal tegmental pontine infarction. Eur Neurol. 1999;41(2):99–102.
11. Tsukita K, Sakamaki-Tsukita H, Suenaga T. Combined abducens and peripheral facial nerve palsy. Intern Med. 2018;57(21):3223–4.
12. Leigh RJ, Zee DS. The neurology of eye movements. 5th ed. Oxford; New York: Oxford University Press; 2015, xx, 1109 pages p.
13. Pham TD, Trobe JD. Selective unidirectional horizontal saccadic paralysis from acute ipsilateral pontine stroke. J Neuroophthalmol. 2017;37(2):159–61.
14. Kato I, Nakamura T, Kanayama R, Aoyagi M. Slow saccades and quick phases of nystagmus after pontine lesions. Acta Otolaryngol Suppl. 1994;511:95–8.
15. Johnston JL, Sharpe JA, Ranalli PJ, Morrow MJ. Oblique misdirection and slowing of vertical saccades after unilateral lesions of the pontine tegmentum. Neurology. 1993;43(11):2238–44.
16. Johnston JL, Sharpe JA, Morrow MJ. Paresis of contralateral smooth pursuit and normal vestibular smooth eye movements after unilateral brainstem lesions. Ann Neurol. 1992;31(5):495–502.
17. Sharpe JA. Neurophysiology and neuroanatomy of smooth pursuit: lesion studies. Brain Cogn. 2008;68(3):241–54.
18. Waespe W. Deficits of smooth-pursuit eye movements in two patients with a lesion in the (para-)floccular or dorsolateral pontine region. Neuro-Ophthalmology. 1992;12(2):91–6.
19. Terao Y, Fukuda H, Shirota Y, Yugeta A, Yoshioka M, Suzuki M, et al. Deterioration of horizontal saccades in progressive supranuclear palsy. Clin Neurophysiol. 2013;124(2):354–63.
20. Ilg UJ, Thier P. The neural basis of smooth pursuit eye movements in the rhesus monkey brain. Brain Cogn. 2008;68(3):229–40.
21. Gaymard B, Pierrot-Deseilligny C, Rivaud S, Velut S. Smooth pursuit eye movement deficits after pontine nuclei lesions in humans. J Neurol Neurosurg Psychiatry. 1993;56(7):799–807.
22. Hanson MR, Hamid MA, Tomsak RL, Chou SS, Leigh RJ. Selective saccadic palsy caused by pontine lesions: clinical, physiological, and pathological correlations. Ann Neurol. 1986;20(2):209–17.

23. Mokri B, Ahlskog JE, Fulgham JR, Matsumoto JY. Syndrome resembling PSP after surgical repair of ascending aorta dissection or aneurysm. Neurology. 2004;62(6):971–3.
24. Nandipati S, Rucker JC, Frucht SJ. Progressive supranuclear palsy-like syndrome after aortic aneurysm repair: a case series. Tremor Other Hyperkinet Mov (N Y). 2013;3:tre-03-201-4686-1.
25. Solomon D, Ramat S, Leigh RJ, Zee D. A quick look at slow saccades after cardiac surgery: where is the lesion? Prog Brain Res. 2008;171:587–90.
26. Solomon D, Ramat S, Tomsak RL, Reich SG, Shin RK, Zee DS, et al. Saccadic palsy after cardiac surgery: characteristics and pathogenesis. Ann Neurol. 2008;63(3):355–65.
27. Tomsak RL, Volpe BT, Stahl JS, Leigh RJ. Saccadic palsy after cardiac surgery: visual disability and rehabilitation. Ann N Y Acad Sci. 2002;956:430–3.
28. Yee RD, Purvin VA. Acquired ocular motor apraxia after aortic surgery. Trans Am Ophthalmol Soc. 2007;105:152–8;discussion 8–9.
29. Horn AK, Bruckner G, Hartig W, Messoudi A. Saccadic omnipause and burst neurons in monkey and human are ensheathed by perineuronal nets but differ in their expression of calcium-binding proteins. J Comp Neurol. 2003;455(3):341–52.
30. Hobohm C, Gunther A, Grosche J, Rossner S, Schneider D, Bruckner G. Decomposition and long-lasting downregulation of extracellular matrix in perineuronal nets induced by focal cerebral ischemia in rats. J Neurosci Res. 2005;80(4):539–48.
31. Eggers SD, Horn AK, Roeber S, Hartig W, Nair G, Reich DS, et al. Saccadic palsy following cardiac surgery: a review and new hypothesis. Ann N Y Acad Sci. 2015;1343:113–9.
32. Strassman A, Evinger C, McCrea RA, Baker RG, Highstein SM. Anatomy and physiology of intracellularly labelled omnipause neurons in the cat and squirrel monkey. Exp Brain Res. 1987;67(2):436–40.
33. Dominguez RO, Bronstein AM. Complete gaze palsy in pontine haemorrhage. J Neurol Neurosurg Psychiatry. 1988;51(1):150–1.
34. Hennerici M, Fromm C. Isolated complete gaze palsy: an unusual ocular movement deficit probably due to a bilateral parapontine reticular formation (PPRF) lesion. Neuro-Ophthalmology. 1981;1(3):165–73.
35. Rufa A, Cerase A, De Santi L, Mandala M, Nuti D, Giorgio A, et al. Impairment of vertical saccades from an acute pontine lesion in multiple sclerosis. J Neuroophthalmol. 2008;28(4):305–7.
36. Slavin ML. A clinicoradiographic correlation of bilateral horizontal gaze palsy and slowed vertical saccades with midline dorsal pontine lesion on magnetic resonance imaging. Am J Ophthalmol. 1986;101(1):118–20.
37. Toyoda K, Hasegawa Y, Yonehara T, Oita J, Yamaguchi T. Bilateral medial medullary infarction with oculomotor disorders. Stroke. 1992;23(11):1657–9.

38. Dell'Osso LF, Robinson DA, Daroff RB. Optokinetic asymmetry in internuclear ophthalmoplegia. Arch Neurol. 1974;31(2):138–9.
39. Gamlin PD, Gnadt JW, Mays LE. Lidocaine-induced unilateral internuclear ophthalmoplegia: effects on convergence and conjugate eye movements. J Neurophysiol. 1989;62(1):82–95.
40. Thömke F, Hopf HC, Breen LA. Slowed abduction saccades in bilateral internuclear ophthalmoplegia. Neuro-Ophthalmology. 1992;12(4):241–6.
41. Stroud MH, Newman NM, Keltner JL, Gay AJ. Abducting nystagmus in the medial longitudinal fasciculus (MLF) syndrome-internuclear ophthalmoplegia (INO). Arch Ophthalmol. 1974;92(1):2–5.
42. Zee DS, Hain TC, Carl JR. Abduction nystagmus in internuclear ophthalmoplegia. Ann Neurol. 1987;21(4):383–8.
43. Baloh RW, Yee RD, Honrubia V. Internuclear ophthalmoplegia. I. Saccades and dissociated nystagmus. Arch Neurol. 1978;35(8):484–9.
44. Buttner-Ennever JA, Horn AK. Pathways from cell groups of the paramedian tracts to the floccular region. Ann N Y Acad Sci. 1996;781:532–40.
45. Brandt TH, Dieterich M. Different types of skew deviation. J Neurol Neurosurg Psychiatry. 1991;54(6):549–50.
46. Zwergal A, Cnyrim C, Arbusow V, Glaser M, Fesl G, Brandt T, et al. Unilateral INO is associated with ocular tilt reaction in pontomesencephalic lesions: INO plus. Neurology. 2008;71(8):590–3.
47. Lee H, Yi HA, Kim HA. Do the paramedian tract neurons in pons take a role as a vertical neural integrator in humans? J Neurol Sci. 2012;321(1–2):107–10.
48. Lee SU, Kim HJ, Kim JS. Evolution of symmetric upbeat into dissociated torsional-upbeat nystagmus in internuclear ophthalmoplegia. Clin Neurol Neurosurg. 2013;115(9):1882–4.
49. Jeong SH, Kim EK, Lee J, Choi KD, Kim JS. Patterns of dissociate torsional-vertical nystagmus in internuclear ophthalmoplegia. Ann N Y Acad Sci. 2011;1233:271–8.
50. Cremer PD, Migliaccio AA, Halmagyi GM, Curthoys IS. Vestibulo-ocular reflex pathways in internuclear ophthalmoplegia. Ann Neurol. 1999;45(4):529–33.
51. Choi SY, Kim HJ, Kim JS. Impaired vestibular responses in internuclear ophthalmoplegia: association and dissociation. Neurology. 2017;89(24):2476–80.
52. Aw ST, Chen L, Todd MJ, Barnett MH, Halmagyi GM. Vestibulo-ocular reflex deficits with medial longitudinal fasciculus lesions. J Neurol. 2017;264(10):2119–29.
53. Wu YT, Cafiero-Chin M, Marques C. Wall-eyed bilateral internuclear ophthalmoplegia: review of pathogenesis, diagnosis, prognosis and management. Clin Exp Optom. 2015;98(1):25–30.
54. Ranalli PJ, Sharpe JA. Vertical vestibulo-ocular reflex, smooth pursuit and eye-head tracking dysfunction in internuclear ophthalmoplegia. Brain. 1988;111(Pt 6):1299–317.

55. Zee DS. Internuclear ophthalmoplegia: pathophysiology and diagnosis. Baillieres Clin Neurol. 1992;1(2):455–70.
56. Takeshige H, Ueno Y, Kamagata K, Sasaki F, Yamashiro K, Tanaka R, et al. Pathways linked to internuclear ophthalmoplegia on diffusion-tensor imaging in a case with midbrain infarction. J Stroke Cerebrovasc Dis. 2016;25(11):2575–9.
57. Xue F, Zhang L, Zhang L, Ying Z, Sha O, Ding Y. One-and-a-half syndrome with its spectrum disorders. Quant Imaging Med Surg. 2017;7(6):691–7.
58. Sharpe JA, Rosenberg MA, Hoyt WF, Daroff RB. Paralytic pontine exotropia. A sign of acute unilateral pontine gaze palsy and internuclear ophthalmoplegia. Neurology. 1974;24(11):1076–81.
59. Komiyama A, Takamatsu K, Johkura K, Hasegawa O, Fukutake T, Hirayama K. Internuclear ophthalmoplegia and contralateral exotropia nonparalytic pontine exotropia and WEBINO syndrome. Neuro-Ophthalmology. 1998;19(1):33–44.
60. Johkura K, Kudo Y, Amano Y, Kikyo H, Imazeki R, Amari K, et al. Gaze palsy and exotropia in internuclear ophthalmoplegia. J Neurol Sci. 2015;353(1–2):158–60.
61. Deleu D, Solheid C, Michotte A, Ebinger G. Dissociated ipsilateral horizontal gaze palsy in one-and-a-half syndrome: a clinicopathologic study. Neurology. 1988;38(8):1278–80.
62. Johnston JL, Sharpe JA. Sparing of the vestibulo-ocular reflex with lesions of the paramedian pontine reticular formation. Neurology. 1989;39(6):876.
63. Kase CS, Maulsby GO, Mohr JP. Partial pontine hematomas. Neurology. 1980;30(6):652–5.
64. Sarwal A, Garewal M, Sahota S, Sivaraman M. Eight-and-a-half syndrome. J Neuroimaging. 2009;19(3):288–90.
65. Marquart C, Strauss C, Alfieri A. Eight-and-a-half syndrome combined with an ipsilateral vertical gaze palsy: a pathophysiological explanation. Clin Neurol Neurosurg. 2013;115(6):767–9.
66. Eggenberger E. Eight-and-a-half syndrome: one-and-a-half syndrome plus cranial nerve VII palsy. J Neuroophthalmol. 1998;18(2):114–6.
67. Li M, Li X, Liu L, Zhu M, Lu D, Wang P. A case report of the rare fifteen-and-a-half syndrome. Medicine (Baltimore). 2019;98(12):e14553.
68. Anderson CA, Sandberg E, Filley CM, Harris SL, Tyler KL. One and one-half syndrome with supranuclear facial weakness: magnetic resonance imaging localization. Arch Neurol. 1999;56(12):1509–11.
69. Cummins G, O'Hare A, Dunne R, Connolly S, O'Rourke K, Lynch T. "Sixteen and a half": a novel pontine neuro-ophthalmological syndrome. J Neurol. 2011;258(7):1347–8.
70. Borgman CJ, Jackson AM. Sixteen-and-a-half syndrome: a variant in the spectrum of Fisher's one-and-a-half syndrome. Clin Exp Optom. 2019;102(1):94–6.

71. Dube M, Dani R, Dubey A, Chouksey D. Twenty-and-a-half syndrome: a case report. J Med Case Rep. 2019;13(1):35.
72. Man BL, Fu YP. 'Twenty-four-and-a-half' syndrome and contralateral hemifacial spasm due to pontine carvernoma. BMJ Case Rep. 2014;2014:bcr2013203268.
73. Satake M, Kira J, Yamada T, Kobayashi T. Raymond syndrome (alternating abducent hemiplegia) caused by a small haematoma at the medial pontomedullary junction. J Neurol Neurosurg Psychiatry. 1995;58(2):261.
74. Megevand P, Pilly B, Delavelle J, Tajouri N, Safran AB, Landis T, et al. Sixth cranial nerve palsy and contralateral hemiparesis (Raymond's syndrome) sparing the face. J Neurol. 2009;256(6):1017–8.
75. Ogawa K, Suzuki Y, Kamei S. Two patients with abducens nerve palsy and crossed hemiplegia (Raymond syndrome). Acta Neurol Belg. 2010;110(3):270–1.
76. Khan M, Naveed S, Haider I, Humayun M, Khan A. Classic Raymond syndrome. J Coll Physicians Surg Pak. 2017;27(3):185–6.
77. Silverman IE, Liu GT, Volpe NJ, Galetta SL. The crossed paralyses. The original brain-stem syndromes of Millard-Gubler, Foville, Weber, and Raymond-Cestan. Arch Neurol. 1995;52(6):635–8.
78. Onbas O, Kantarci M, Alper F, Karaca L, Okur A. Millard-Gubler syndrome: MR findings. Neuroradiology. 2005;47(1):35–7.
79. Krasnianski M, Wendt M, Muller T, Zierz S. Raymond-Cestan syndrome in pontine ischemia. Clin Neurol Neurosurg. 2007;109(9):834–5.

Eye Movements and Vestibular Dysfunction: Lesions of Midbrain

9

Several midbrain structures control eye movements during gaze-shifts and gaze-holding. This chapter outlines key functional impairments in eye movements and vestibular function that are seen after lesions affecting midbrain structures (Table 9.1).

Rostral Interstitial Nucleus of the Medial Longitudinal Fasciculus (riMLF)

The riMLF is a wing-shaped mesencephalic structure, dorsomedial to red nucleus, at the level of superior colliculus (Fig. 9.1). The Fig. 9.1 demonstrates the simplified cross sectional view of the rostral midbrain; the riMLF is on the rostral part of MLF. The riMLF houses the burst neurons for vertical and torsional eye movements, and it sends collaterals to the motor neurons supplying yoked muscle pair [1, 2]. As a result, riMLF lesion typically leads to conjugate gaze deficit. The riMLF project to the motor neurons for bilateral elevators (the superior rectus and inferior oblique) and to the ipsilateral depressor muscles (inferior rectus and superior oblique) [1]. Unilateral riMLF lesions could affect downward saccades, and the quick phase of ipsilateral cyclorotation [3–6]. The riMLF is responsible for the quick phase of extorting ipsilateral eye and intorting contralateral eye. Consequently,

A. Shaikh, F. Wang, *Eye Movements in the Critical Care Setting*,
https://doi.org/10.1007/978-3-030-70221-2_9

Table 9.1 Ocular motor dysfunction in midbrain lesions

RiMLF (unilateral)	Variable defect of downward saccades No or minimal defect of upward saccades Loss of ipsitorsional quick phase Static, contralesional torsional deviation (top pole of the eyeball deviated away from the lesion side) Contralesional torsional nystagmus (top pole of the eyeball beating contralateral to the lesion side)
RiMLF (bilateral)	Profound vertical saccades abnormalities, especially downward saccades Preserved vertical gaze holding, VOR, pursuit and horizontal eye movements
INC (unilateral)	Ocular tilt reactions Ipsilesional torsional nystagmus
INC (bilateral)	Restrictions of all vertical conjugate eye movements, except for saccades
Posterior Commissure	Impairment of all vertical eye movements, with loss of vertical gaze holding Convergence disorders Convergence-retraction nystagmus Collier's sign Pupils are mid-dilated and may have light-near dissociation
Superior Colliculus	Increased latency and accuracy on contralateral saccades Impaired saccades learning
CN III Palsy	Complete: Ipsilateral eye deviated "down and out" Contralateral superior rectus paresis Mild bilateral ptosis Superior Rectus Subnucleus: Bilateral superior rectus palsy Central Caudal Subnucleus: Bilateral ptosis or "plus-minus" lid syndrome Medial Rectus Subnucleus: Medial rectus palsy Inferior Rectus and Inferior Oblique Subnucleus: Inferior rectus palsy and inferior oblique palsy Oculomotor Internuclear Neurons: Contralateral abduction weakness and esotropia Vertical one-and-a-half syndrome
CN IV Palsy	Ipsilateral hypertropia Head tilts away from the lesion side

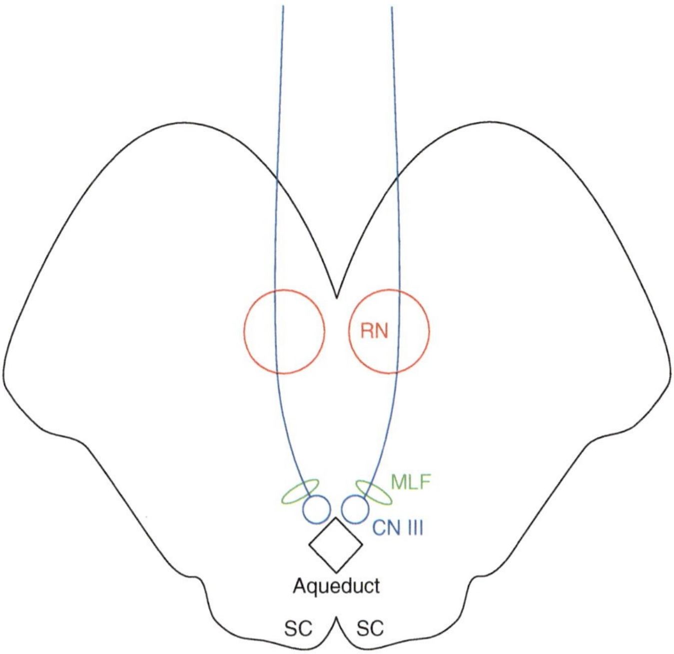

Fig. 9.1 The schematic illustrates the cross-sectional view of the midbrain. *RN* red nucleus, *MLF* medial longitudinal fasciculus, *CN III* oculomotor nucleus, *SC* superior colliculus

the riMLF lesion causes tonic cyclodeviation (ocular torsion) towards to side contralateral to the lesion [7, 8]. It is noteworthy that riMLF resides in a very compact part of the brain, and they are close to midline; hence bilateral riMLF lesions are more common clinically. Bilateral riMLF lesions can impair downward saccades [9, 10]. However, complete vertical saccadic deficit in conjunction with impairment of quick phase of cyclorotation is also not uncommon with mesencephalic lesion involving bilateral riMLF. The riMLF lesion can also impair vertical smooth pursuit and vestibulo-ocular reflex. When this happens, it usually suggests the lesion has extended to adjacent area and the interstitial nucleus of Cajal [11].

Interstitial Nucleus of Cajal (INC)

The INC is the neural integrator for the vertical gaze holding. The nucleus receives the pulse of eye velocity signal (from the burst neurons) and converts it into a steady state signal keeping the eyes steady [12, 13]. The INC projections travel through the posterior commissure or via ipsilateral projections to reach ocular motoneurons [14, 15]. The unilateral INC lesion is responsible for the ocular tilt reaction and ipsilesional torsional nystagmus with quick phase towards the lesion side. To compare and contrast, INC lesion produces ipsilesional torsional nystagmus whereas riMLF injury leads to contralesional torsional nystagmus [8, 16, 17]. Bilateral INC lesions restricts conjugate vertical eye movements other than saccades which are controlled by the riMLF [12].

Posterior Commissure and Nucleus of the Posterior Commissure

Lesions of posterior commissure have many eponyms such as dorsal midbrain syndrome, Parinaud's syndrome, Koeber-Salus-Elschig syndrome, pretectal syndrome, and Sylvian aqueduct syndrome [18]. The posterior commissure lesions present with constellation of symptoms, such as limited upward eye movements, dissociation of lid and eye movements, disturbance of downward and vergence eye movements, square-wave jerks, see-saw nystagmus, skew deviation, ocular tilt reaction, and pupil abnormalities. Selective upgaze deficits from posterior commissure lesion can mimic bilateral INC lesions, however, projections from INC to depressor muscles do not cross via posterior commissure. As a result, the downward eye movements are relatively spared in posterior commissure lesion [14].

The group of neurons within posterior commissure, called the nucleus of posterior commissure, are connected with the contralateral riMLF, contralateral INC, and the "M" group nuclei [19, 20]. Impairment of the "M" group nuclei manifests as transient eyelid lag with downward gaze shifts, but without sustained eyelid retraction [21]. Such dissociation, the Collier's sign or "tucked lid" sign, is often seen with an abrupt increase in the intracranial pressure, which can be frequently observed in critically ill patients. It is characterized by tonic downward deviation of the eyes, "setting-sun" sign. Tonic upward gaze deviation of eyes was also reported in critically ill patients with midbrain lesions and following hypoxic ischemic injuries [22–24]. It is believed that disinhibition of the cerebellar projections due to Purkinje neuron injuries leads to such deficit [24, 25].

Vergence abnormality is not uncommon with posterior commissure lesions. In some instances, the convergence is paralyzed, while in others there is excessive convergence leading to convergence "spasm". The convergence spasm often presents as slowed abduction velocity but normal adduction, or even complete disability to abduct the eyes. It might mimic abducens palsy, hence called "pseudo"abducens palsy [26–28]. Moreover, normally interneurons within oculomotor nucleus would also send excitatory projections to contralateral abducens nucleus to facilitate abduction. Injury to these projections also explain "pseudo"abducens palsy [29–31].

Convergence retraction nystagmus is associated with structural lesions affecting the posterior commissure or pretectal area [32–37]. It is believed that convergence retraction nystagmus is due to asynchronous (disconjugate) horizontal saccades when upward quick phase are warranted. The convergence retraction nystagmus is also considered to be a primary vergence disorder [38]. The convergence is typically evident during large upward saccades. The pupillary responses are frequently impaired, the pupils have better reaction to near stimuli than to the light, i.e., "light-near dissociation".

Superior Colliculus

Superior colliculus acts as a hub communicating between the cerebral cortex and the basal ganglia with brainstem motor and premotor nuclei for ocular motor control (Fig. 9.2). It is typically

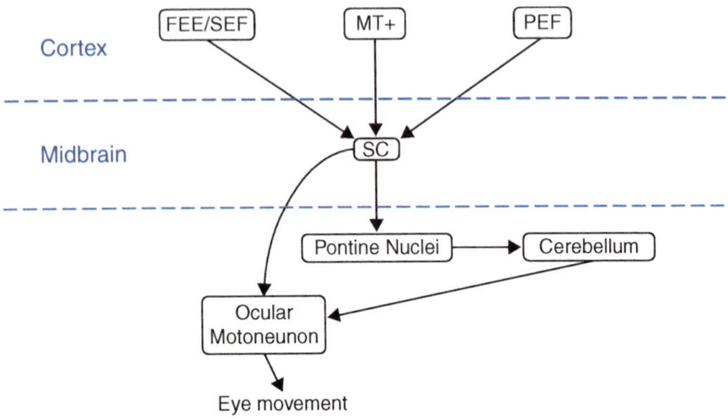

Fig. 9.2 Illustration of the simplified connections between each cortical eye field and final pathway. Superior colliculus acts as a hub to relay signals from supratentorial commands

uncommon to get an isolated superior colliculus lesion; however, it is frequent to have superior colliculus damage in addition to other ocular motor nuclei. Selective lesion of the superior colliculus, in humans, can cause persistent limitation of upward gaze, implying pretectal damage, with preserved horizontal eye movements [39].

Oculomotor Nerve Palsy

The oculomotor nerve (IIIrd nerve) innervates the ipsilateral medial rectus, inferior rectus, and inferior oblique; contralateral superior rectus; and bilateral levator palpebrae. The parasympathetic fibers from Edinger Westphal nucleus also join the IIIrd nerve to innervate the ciliary body. A complete IIIrd nerve palsy manifests as ipsilateral eye in a down and out orientation [40]. However incomplete IIIrd nerve palsy is more common in clinical practice [41].

Nuclear IIIrd Nerve Palsy

Isolated IIIrd nucleus lesion is rare, but can be seen in lacunar infarcts due to the occlusion of the long branches of paramedian perforators [42]. A complete IIIrd nucleus lesion can lead to an ipsilateral IIIrd nerve palsy, contralateral superior rectus weakness, and bilateral mild ptosis.

The IIIrd nucleus is divided into many subregions. The one for superior rectus, if involved, causes bilateral superior rectus palsy [43–45]. The involvement of the central caudal subnucleus presents with bilateral ptosis via bilateral levator palpebrae involvement [46–51]. "Plus-minus" lid syndrome is characterized by ipsilateral ptosis and contralateral upper eyelid retraction and this can be observed after central caudal subnucleus injury [52–56]. It is postulated that the contralateral lid retraction is caused by disinhibition of lid activation due to lesions involving "M" group neurons projections [56]. In such case, the lesion is more likely to involve the fascicles of caudal central subnucleus rather than the subnucleus itself. At times, one ptotic eyelid plus the other retracted eyelid could be seen in myasthenia gravis sometimes, which is called pseudo-plus-minus lid syndrome [57]. The passive elevation of the ptotic eyelid will abolish the contralateral eyelid retraction in myasthenia due to the Hering's law of equal innervation, whereas in true plus-minus lid syndrome, lid retraction is not influenced [58, 59]. The medial rectus subnuclei are in two different locations within the IIIrd nucleus, so it is highly unlikely to have isolated medial rectus weakness from nuclear IIIrd nerve palsy [60]. The pupillary defect suggests rostral IIIrd nuclear lesion and such lesion is dorsal to the Edinger-Westphal nucleus [61]. Oculomotor internuclear interneurons within IIIrd nucleus project to the contralateral abducens nucleus [29–31]. Impairment of these interneurons lead to contralesional abduction deficit along with esotropia. The loss of downward movements and selective loss of upward movements in one eye; or the bilateral loss of upward movements and selective loss of downward movement in one eye is the basis for the vertical one-and-a-half syndrome [62–65]. The vertical one-and-a-half syndrome is due to lesions extending to the INC, riMLF, posterior commissure and the IIIrd nucleus or its nerve fascicles.

Fascicular IIIrd Nerve Palsy

The fascicles of the IIIrd nerve emerge through the entire dimension of the IIIrd nucleus. The topographical distribution of different muscle fibers varies. Most medially, pupil fibers are rostral and inferior rectus fibers are caudal. Then, inferior rectus is rostral, medial rectus is middle, and levator palpebrare is caudal. Most laterally, the inferior oblique is rostral and superior rectus is caudal [42, 66–69] (Fig. 9.3). The Fig. 9.3 demonstrates a cross section view of IIIrd nerve. As IIIrd nerve exits the midbrain, it travels through the subarachnoid space, passing by the circle of Willis, having the basilar artery on the medial, posterior cerebral artery above, and superior cerebellar artery below the nerve. The

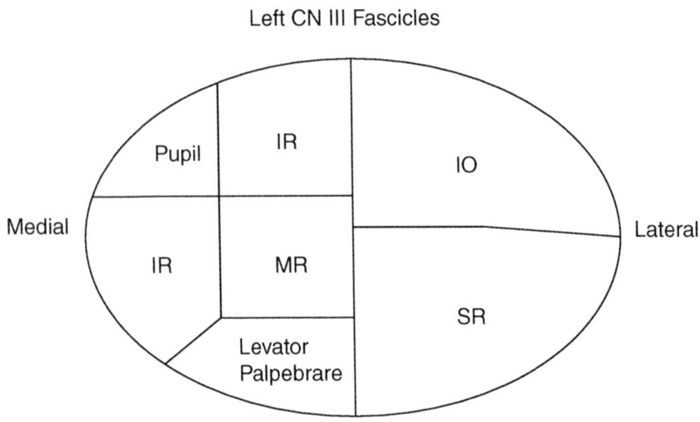

Fig. 9.3 Schematic cross section view of left IIIrd nerve fascicle. Most medially, rostral to caudal is pupil and inferior rectus (IR). Then inferior rectus (IR) followed by medial rectus (MR) and levator palpebrare. Most laterally, from rostral to caudal is inferior oblique (IO) and superior rectus (SR)

strategic anatomical relationship between the IIIrd nerve and the blood vessels are the basis for the oculomotor palsies in patients with various forms of aneurysms. Typically aneurysms involve pupil fibers, but in acute phases the pupillary reflex may be spared [70–73]. Temporal lobe herniation also can compress the IIIrd neve against the tentorial edge, petroclinoid ligament or clivus [74, 75]. In those with herniation, the IIIrd nerve can be stretched due to the midbrain displacement. Just as seen in patients with compressive aneurysms, the pupil fibers are affected first, leading to mydriasis of the ipsilateral eye. Fixed and dilated ipsilateral pupil is then followed by extraocular muscle weakness.

The IIIrd nerve palsy is also associated with the microvascular infarction caused by diabetes or hypertension, occasionally related to collagen vascular disease, giant cell arteritis or end-stage renal disease [76–79]. In such cases the pupillary reflex remains normal or patients may have mild anisocoria [80]. The patients usually complain of pain preceding the ophthalmoparesis, but the pain disappears when the diplopia or ptosis develops. The onset of diplopia is generally sudden, but the extraocular muscles palsy may evolve and develop for up to a few weeks, and the recovery is usually achieved within 3 months [81, 82].

Trochlear Nerve Palsy

The fascicles of the trochlear nerve (IVth nerve) exit the midbrain from its dorsal aspect and then crosses the midline. The cumbersome course of this nerve is the reason for its frequent involvement in traumatic diplopia where the subjects develop obliquely spaced double vision especially while looking down [83, 84].

The clinical signs of IVth nerve palsy include hypertropia of the affected eye and the (compensatory) head tilt away from the lesion side. Bielschowsky head-tilt test, which can reliably differentiate the IVth nerve palsy from skew deviation, is based on the principle that hypertropia is maximized as the head tilts towards the lesion side and minimized when tilting to the opposite site. The patients with IVth nerve palsy may have normal velocities of the downward saccades, but they may be hypometric [85].

Midbrain Stroke Syndromes

The strategic locations of IIIrd and IVth nerve, corresponding nuclei, and premotor structures such as INC and riMLF in midbrain forms the background for different stroke syndrome. Even small lacunar infarct can involve more than one areas for ocular motor control; and minor shift in the location of the lesion can present with completely different symptomatology. The midbrain stroke syndromes are known with various eponyms (Table 9.2).

Weber's Syndrome

The Weber's syndrome is comprised of ipsilateral IIIrd nerve palsy and contralateral hemiparesis (Fig. 9.4). The underlying mechanism is that the stroke at the region where oculomotor nerve passes through the cerebral peduncle causes combination of IIIrd nerve palsy and contralateral weakness [86].

Claude's Syndrome

The Claude's syndrome consists of ipsilateral IIIrd nerve palsy, contralateral ataxia, asynergy and dysdiadochokinesis [87–90]

Table 9.2 Midbrain stroke syndromes

Weber's Syndrome	Ipsilateral CN III palsy Contralateral hemiparesis
Claude's Syndrome	Ipsilateral CN III palsy Contralateral ataxia
Benedikt's Syndrome	Ipsilateral CN III palsy Contralateral ataxia Contralateral extrapyramidal signs (tremor)
Nothnagel's Syndrome	Ipsilateral CN III palsy Contralateral ataxia Supranuclear gaze palsy

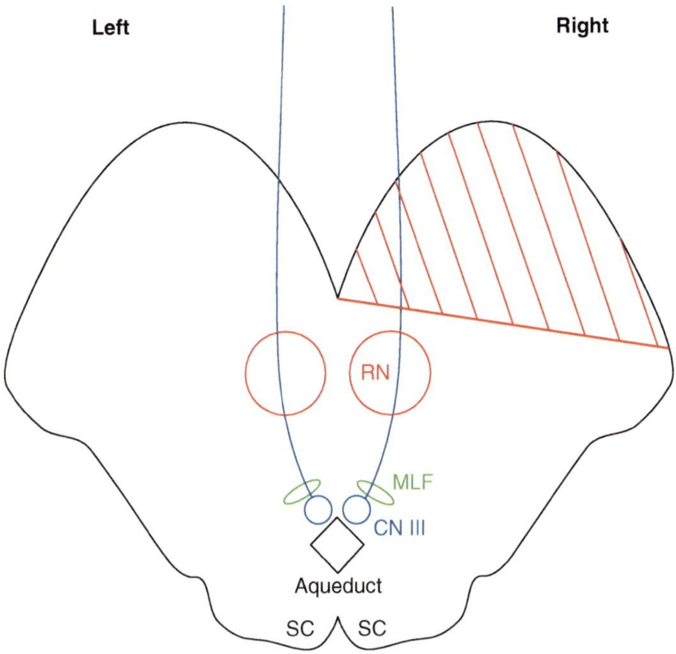

Fig. 9.4 A schematic of right-sided Weber's syndrome. The lesion involves right sided cerebral peduncle, IIIrd nerve fibers leading to left hemiparesis and right IIIrd nerve palsy

(Fig. 9.5). The lesion involves IIIrd nerve fascicles, red nucleus and superior cerebellar peduncle. It is noteworthy that the cerebral peduncle is spared.

Benedikt's Syndrome

The patients with Benedikt's syndrome have ipsilateral IIIrd nerve palsy, as well as contralateral ataxia and tremor [54]. The Benedikt syndrome is analogous to the Claude's syndrome, but with relatively milder involvement.

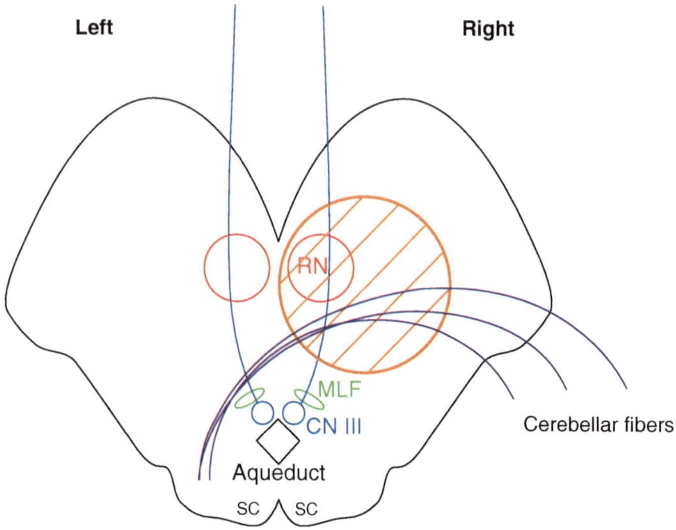

Fig. 9.5 Schematic depicting right Claude's syndrome. The lesion involves right red nucleus, cerebellar fibers crossing over from left side and right IIIrd nerve. Such lesion causes right IIIrd nerve palsy, left-sided ataxia

Nothnagel's Syndrome

Nothnagel's syndrome is a combination of nuclear IIIrd palsy, supranuclear gaze palsy, and contralateral ataxia [91, 92] (Fig. 9.6). Lesion of Nothnagel's syndrome is more dorsal, involving the oculomotor nucleus, superior cerebellar peduncle and posterior commissure. Frequently, because of larger involvement, vertical one-and-a-half syndrome can be one of the manifestations.

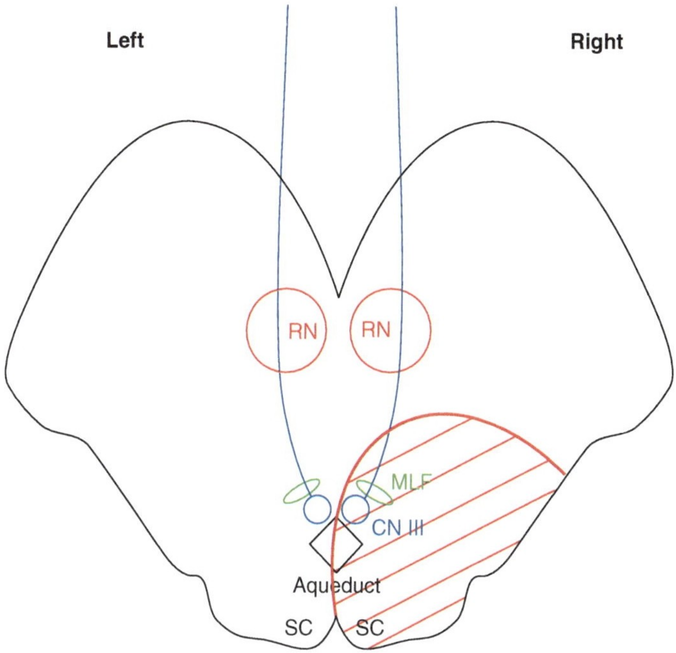

Fig. 9.6 Schematic of right Nothnagel's syndrome. The lesion involves right IIIrd nucleus, superior cerebellar peduncle and pretectal plate

Summary

In this chapter, we reviewed the important structures within midbrain concerned with eye movements. Rostral interstitial medial longitudinal fasciculus (RiMLF) acts as the vertical saccade generator. Unilateral RiMLF injury leads to ipsilateral defect of downward saccades, whereas bilateral lesions cause profound vertical saccades abnormalities. Interstitial nucleus of Cajal (INC) is known as the neural integrator for the vertical and torsional gaze. Lesion of unilateral INC leads to ocular tilt reaction and ipsilesional torsional nystagmus, whereas bilateral lesion causes loss of all vertical eye movements except for saccades. Lesions involving posterior commissure are commonly known as Parinaud's syndrome. Patients manifest with constellation of symptoms – impairment of all vertical eye movements, convergence-retraction nystagmus, convergence disorders, collier's sign and mid-size nonreactive pupils. The superior colliculus, sitting in the dorsal aspect of the midbrain, is a relay station for vision pathway. Injury of superior colliculus leads to impaired saccade learning and increased latency and decreased accuracy of saccades. The nuclei of oculomotor nerve (CN III) and trochlear nerve (CN IV) are also located in the midbrain. Injury of CN III can cause a wide range of presentation ranging from complete CN III palsy – "down and out" deviation of ipsilateral eye with nonreactive pupils – or palsy of one of the specific muscles. CN IV palsy could cause hypertropia of the ipsilateral eye and head tilting towards contralateral side. Last but not the least, common midbrain stroke syndromes manifest with eye movement abnormalities. These include Weber's syndrome, Claude's syndrome, Benedikt's syndrome and Nothnagel's syndrome.

References

1. Moschovakis AK, Scudder CA, Highstein SM. A structural basis for Hering's law: projections to extraocular motoneurons. Science. 1990;248(4959):1118–9.
2. Teske SA, Kersten RC, Devoto MH, Kulwin DR. Hering's law and eyebrow position. Ophthalmic Plast Reconstr Surg. 1998;14(2):105–6.
3. Ahlfeld J, Mustari M, Horn AK. Sources of calretinin inputs to motoneurons of extraocular muscles involved in upgaze. Ann N Y Acad Sci. 2011;1233:91–9.
4. Zeeh C, Hess BJ, Horn AK. Calretinin inputs are confined to motoneurons for upward eye movements in monkey. J Comp Neurol. 2013;521(14):3154–66.

5. Riordan-Eva P, Faldon M, Buttner-Ennever JA, Gass A, Bronstein AM, Gresty MA. Abnormalities of torsional fast phase eye movements in unilateral rostral midbrain disease. Neurology. 1996;47(1):201–7.
6. Leigh RJ, Seidman SH, Grant MP, Hanna JP. Loss of ipsidirectional quick phases of torsional nystagmus with a unilateral midbrain lesion. J Vestib Res. 1993;3(2):115–21.
7. Buuttner U, Buuttner-Ennever JA, Rambold H, Helmchen C. The contribution of midbrain circuits in the control of gaze. Ann N Y Acad Sci. 2002;956:99–110.
8. Helmchen C, Rambold H, Kempermann U, Buttner-Ennever JA, Buttner U. Localizing value of torsional nystagmus in small midbrain lesions. Neurology. 2002;59(12):1956–64.
9. Pierrot-Deseilligny CH, Chain F, Gray F, Serdaru M, Escourolle R, Lhermitte F. Parinaud's syndrome: electro-oculographic and anatomical analyses of six vascular cases with deductions about vertical gaze organization in the premotor structures. Brain. 1982;105(Pt 4):667–96.
10. Mossman SS, Bronstein AM, Gresty MA, Kendall B, Rudge P. Convergence nystagmus associated with Arnold-Chiari malformation. Arch Neurol. 1990;47(3):357–9.
11. Sharpe JA, Kim JS. Midbrain disorders of vertical gaze: a quantitative re-evaluation. Ann N Y Acad Sci. 2002;956:143–54.
12. Helmchen C, Rambold H, Fuhry L, Buttner U. Deficits in vertical and torsional eye movements after uni- and bilateral muscimol inactivation of the interstitial nucleus of Cajal of the alert monkey. Exp Brain Res. 1998;119(4):436–52.
13. Crawford JD, Cadera W, Vilis T. Generation of torsional and vertical eye position signals by the interstitial nucleus of Cajal. Science. 1991;252(5012):1551–3.
14. Horn AK, Helmchen C, Wahle P. GABAergic neurons in the rostral mesencephalon of the macaque monkey that control vertical eye movements. Ann N Y Acad Sci. 2003;1004:19–28.
15. Kokkoroyannis T, Scudder CA, Balaban CD, Highstein SM, Moschovakis AK. Anatomy and physiology of the primate interstitial nucleus of Cajal I. efferent projections. J Neurophysiol. 1996;75(2):725–39.
16. Ohashi T, Fukushima K, Chin S, Harada T, Yoshida K, Akino M, et al. Ocular tilt reaction with vertical eye movement palsy caused by localized unilateral midbrain lesion. J Neuroophthalmol. 1998;18(1):40–2.
17. Oh SY, Choi KD, Shin BS, Seo MW, Kim YH, Kim JS. Paroxysmal ocular tilt reactions after mesodiencephalic lesions: report of two cases and review of the literature. J Neurol Sci. 2009;277(1–2):98–102.
18. Feroze KB, Patel BC. Parinaud Syndrome. Treasure Island: StatPearls; 2019.
19. Buttner-Ennever JA, Horn AKE, Olszewski J. Olszewski and Baxter's Cytoarchitecture of the human brainstem. 3rd, revised and extended edition ed. Basel; New York: Karger; 2014, xii, 290 pages p.

20. Schmidtke K, Buttner-Ennever JA. Nervous control of eyelid function. A review of clinical, experimental and pathological data. Brain. 1992;115(Pt 1):227–47.
21. Galetta SL, Raps EC, Liu GT, Saito NG, Kline LB. Eyelid lag without eyelid retraction in pretectal disease. J Neuroophthalmol. 1996;16(2): 96–8.
22. Barontini F, Simonetti C, Ferranini F, Sita D. Persistent upward eye deviation report of two cases. Neuro-Ophthalmology. 1983;3(4):217–24.
23. Keane JR. Sustained upgaze in coma. Ann Neurol. 1981;9(4):409–12.
24. Johkura K, Komiyama A, Kuroiwa Y. Vertical conjugate eye deviation in postresuscitation coma. Ann Neurol. 2004;56(6):878–81.
25. Lankford J, Butler IJ. Transient tonic upgaze deviation: a neuro-ophthalmological complication of acute cerebellitis. J Child Neurol. 2013;28(7):942–4.
26. Pullicino P, Lincoff N, Truax BT. Abnormal vergence with upper brainstem infarcts: pseudoabducens palsy. Neurology. 2000;55(3):352–8.
27. Thurtell MJ, Leigh RJ, Halmagyi GM. Monocular ophthalmoplegia and partial supranuclear vertical gaze palsy due to unilateral paramedian rostral midbrain infarction. J Neurol. 2009;256(4):664–6.
28. Kaas BM, Zee DS, Kheradmand A, Gold DR. Midbrain infarction resulting in bilateral pseudoabducens palsies. Neurologist. 2017;22(3):72–6.
29. Maciewicz R, Phipps BS. The oculomotor internuclear pathway: a double retrograde labeling study. Brain Res. 1983;262(1):1–8.
30. Clendaniel RA, Mays LE. Characteristics of antidromically identified oculomotor internuclear neurons during vergence and versional eye movements. J Neurophysiol. 1994;71(3):1111–27.
31. Buttner-Ennever JA. The extraocular motor nuclei: organization and functional neuroanatomy. Prog Brain Res. 2006;151:95–125.
32. Pasik P, Pasik T, Bender MB. The pretectal syndrome in monkeys. I. Disturbances of gaze and body posture. Brain. 1969;92(3):521–34.
33. Pasik T, Pasik P, Bender MB. The pretectal syndrome in monkeys. II. Spontaneous and induced nystagmus, and "lightning" eye movements. Brain. 1969;92(4):871–84.
34. Gay AJ, Brodkey J, Miller JE. Convergence retraction nystagums. An electromyographic study. Arch Ophthalmol. 1963;70:456–61.
35. Herishanu Y. Convergence nystagmus in brain stem tuberculoma. Ophthalmologica. 1971;163(2):98–101.
36. Sato Y, Maehara F, Utsunomiya H, Hayashi T, Moritaka K, Kaji M. Convergence and retraction nystagmus in hydrocephalus due to shunt malfunction. Kurume Med J. 1983;30(4):125–8.
37. Luda E, Sicuro L, Albera R, Roberto C, De Lucchi R. Retraction-convergence nystagmus: clinical and radiological study of 4 cases of vascular origin. Ital J Neurol Sci. 1992;13(2):119–24.
38. Rambold H, Kompf D, Helmchen C. Convergence retraction nystagmus: a disorder of vergence? Ann Neurol. 2001;50(5):677–81.

39. Heywood SRG. Long-term oculomotor consequences of unilateral colliculectomy in man. In: Lennerstrand G, Bach-y-Rita P, editors. Basic mechanisms of ocular motility and their clinical implications. Oxford: Pergamon; 1986. p. 561–4.
40. Johnston AC, Pratt-Johnson JA. The ocular sequelae of third cranial nerve palsy. Can Med Assoc J. 1963;89:871–3.
41. Biousse V, Newman NJ. Third nerve palsies. Semin Neurol. 2000;20(1):55–74.
42. Vitosevic Z, Marinkovic S, Cetkovic M, Stimec B, Todorovic V, Kanjuh V, et al. Intramesencephalic course of the oculomotor nerve fibers: microanatomy and possible clinical significance. Anat Sci Int. 2013;88(2): 70–82.
43. Gaymard B, Larmande P, de Toffol B, Autret A. Reversible nuclear oculomotor nerve paralysis. Caused by a primary mesencephalic hemorrhage. Eur Neurol. 1990;30(3):128–31.
44. Bryan JS, Hamed LM. Levator-sparing nuclear oculomotor palsy. Clinical and magnetic resonance imaging findings. J Clin Neuroophthalmol. 1992;12(1):26–30.
45. Bienfang DC. Crossing axons in the third nerve nucleus. Investig Ophthalmol. 1975;14(12):927–31.
46. Conway VH, Rozdilsky B, Schneider RJ, Sundaram M. Isolated bilateral complete ptosis. Can J Ophthalmol. 1983;18(1):37–40.
47. Iwanaga K, Kinoshita I, Ohe N. Brainstem ptosis (midbrain ptosis) associated with mesencephalic hemorrhage. Rinsho Shinkeigaku. 1990;30(7):793–5.
48. Martin TJ, Corbett JJ, Babikian PV, Crawford SC, Currier RD. Bilateral ptosis due to mesencephalic lesions with relative preservation of ocular motility. J Neuroophthalmol. 1996;16(4):258–63.
49. Kao YF, Lan MY, Chou MS, Chen WH. Intracranial fatigable ptosis. J Neuroophthalmol. 1999;19(4):257–9.
50. In YS, Shin SY, Song BJ. A case of bilateral oculomotor nuclear palsy. Korean J Ophthalmol. 2003;17(1):67–70.
51. Maranhao-Filho P, Pires ME. Metastasis to the unilateral oculomotor nucleus complex: case report. Arq Neuropsiquiatr. 2006;64(2B):520–2.
52. Gaymard B, Lafitte C, Gelot A, de Toffol B. Plus-minus lid syndrome. J Neurol Neurosurg Psychiatry. 1992;55(9):846–8.
53. Porta-Etessam J, Benito-Leon J, Berbel A, Martinez A. Plus minus lid syndrome without ophthalmoplegia. Eur J Neurol. 1999;6(1):107.
54. Akdal G, Kutluk K, Men S, Yaka E. Benedikt and "plus-minus lid" syndromes arising from posterior cerebral artery branch occlusion. J Neurol Sci. 2005;228(1):105–7.
55. Kotwal VS, Shenoy VV, Joshi SR, Aklujkar AP, Nadkami NA, Shetty K, et al. Plus minus lid syndrome with ataxia. J Assoc Physicians India. 2005;53:908–9.

56. Alsherbini K, Kapadia K, Sattin JA. A rare midbrain infarction presenting with plus-minus lid syndrome with ataxia: a case report. J Med Case Rep. 2011;5:525.
57. Bandini F. Pseudo plus-minus lid syndrome. Arch Neurol. 2009;66(5):668–9.
58. Averbuch-Heller L, Poonyathalang A, von Maydell RD, Remler BF. Hering's law for eyelids: still valid. Neurology. 1995;45(9):1781–3.
59. Chen AD, Lai YW, Lai HT, Huang SH, Lee SS, Chang KP, et al. The impact of Hering's law in blepharoptosis: literature review. Ann Plast Surg. 2016;76(Suppl 1):S96–100.
60. Al-Sofiani M, Lee KP. Isolated medial rectus nuclear palsy as a rare presentation of midbrain infarction. Am J Case Rep. 2015;16:715–8.
61. Horn AK, Eberhorn A, Hartig W, Ardeleanu P, Messoudi A, Buttner-Ennever JA. Perioculomotor cell groups in monkey and man defined by their histochemical and functional properties: reappraisal of the Edinger-Westphal nucleus. J Comp Neurol. 2008;507(3):1317–35.
62. Deleu D, Buisseret T, Ebinger G. Vertical one-and-a-half syndrome. Supranuclear downgaze paralysis with monocular elevation palsy. Arch Neurol. 1989;46(12):1361–3.
63. Hommel M, Bogousslavsky J. The spectrum of vertical gaze palsy following unilateral brainstem stroke. Neurology. 1991;41(8):1229–34.
64. Deleu D, Imam YZ, Mesraoua B, Salem KY. Vertical one-and-a-half syndrome with contralesional pseudo-abducens palsy in a patient with thalamomesencephalic stroke. J Neurol Sci. 2012;312(1–2):180–3.
65. Sato K, Takahashi Y, Matsumoto N, Yunoki T, Takemoto M, Hishikawa N, et al. Rare valiant vertical one-and-a-half syndrome without ipsilateral upward gaze palsy in a patient with thalamomesencephalic stroke. Neurol Clin Neurosci. 2018;6(5):133–5.
66. Ksiazek SM, Repka MX, Maguire A, Harbour RC, Savino PJ, Miller NR, et al. Divisional oculomotor nerve paresis caused by intrinsic brainstem disease. Ann Neurol. 1989;26(6):714–8.
67. Castro O, Johnson LN, Mamourian AC. Isolated inferior oblique paresis from brain-stem infarction. Perspective on oculomotor fascicular organization in the ventral midbrain tegmentum. Arch Neurol. 1990;47(2):235–7.
68. Schwartz TH, Lycette CA, Yoon SS, Kargman DE. Clinicoradiographic evidence for oculomotor fascicular anatomy. J Neurol Neurosurg Psychiatry. 1995;59(3):338.
69. Purvin V. Photo essay. Isolated fascicular third nerve palsy. J Neuroophthalmol. 2010;30(3):263–5.
70. Kissel JT, Burde RM, Klingele TG, Zeiger HE. Pupil-sparing oculomotor palsies with internal carotid-posterior communicating artery aneurysms. Ann Neurol. 1983;13(2):149–54.
71. Ajtai B, Fine EJ, Lincoff N. Pupil-sparing, painless compression of the oculomotor nerve by expanding basilar artery aneurysm: a case of ocular pseudomyasthenia. Arch Neurol. 2004;61(9):1448–50.

72. Motoyama Y, Nonaka J, Hironaka Y, Park YS, Nakase H. Pupil-sparing oculomotor nerve palsy caused by upward compression of a large posterior communicating artery aneurysm. Case report. Neurol Med Chir (Tokyo). 2012;52(4):202–5.
73. Keane JR. Aneurysms and third nerve palsies. Ann Neurol. 1983;14(6):696–7.
74. Posner JB, Plum F. Plum and Posner's diagnosis of stupor and coma. 4th ed. Oxford; New York: Oxford University Press; 2007, xiv, 401 pages p.
75. Zhang CH, DeSouza RM, Kho JS, Vundavalli S, Critchley G. Kernohan-Woltman notch phenomenon: a review article. Br J Neurosurg. 2017;31(2):159–66.
76. Davies GE, Shakir RA. Giant cell arteritis presenting as oculomotor nerve palsy with pupillary dilatation. Postgrad Med J. 1994;70(822):298–9.
77. Nakamagoe K, Yanagiha H, Miyake Z, Kondo Y, Hiyama T, Ishii A, et al. Monocular oculomotor nerve disorder manifesting as cranial neuropathy in systemic lupus erythematosus. Intern Med. 2018;57(23):3445–9.
78. Greco D, Gambina F, Maggio F. Ophthalmoplegia in diabetes mellitus: a retrospective study. Acta Diabetol. 2009;46(1):23–6.
79. Komine N, Ohnari K, Murakami M, Kawata K, Suzuka K, Nakamata T. Ischemic ocular motor nerve palsy in three patients with end-stage renal disease. J UOEH. 2006;28(1):57–64.
80. Jacobson DM. Pupil involvement in patients with diabetes-associated oculomotor nerve palsy. Arch Ophthalmol. 1998;116(6):723–7.
81. Jacobson DM, Broste SK. Early progression of ophthalmoplegia in patients with ischemic oculomotor nerve palsies. Arch Ophthalmol. 1995;113(12):1535–7.
82. Capo H, Warren F, Kupersmith MJ. Evolution of oculomotor nerve palsies. J Clin Neuroophthalmol. 1992;12(1):21–5.
83. Schworm HD, Horstmann S, Ring T, Boergen KP. Changes in subjective cyclodeviation and objective cycloposition after modified Harada-Ito operation in acquired trochlear paralysis. Klin Monatsbl Augenheilkd. 1998;212(4):207–11.
84. Roh YR, Hwang JM. Comparison of subjective and objective torsion in patients with acquired unilateral superior oblique muscle palsy. Br J Ophthalmol. 2011;95(11):1583–7.
85. Tian S, Lennerstrand G. Vertical saccadic velocity and force development in superior oblique palsy. Vis Res. 1994;34(13):1785–98.
86. Silverman IE, Liu GT, Volpe NJ, Galetta SL. The crossed paralyses. The original brain-stem syndromes of Millard-Gubler, Foville, Weber, and Raymond-Cestan. Arch Neurol. 1995;52(6):635–8.
87. Seo SW, Heo JH, Lee KY, Shin WC, Chang DI, Kim SM, et al. Localization of Claude's syndrome. Neurology. 2001;57(12):2304–7.

88. Broadley SA, Taylor J, Waddy HM, Thompson PD. The clinical and MRI correlate of ischaemia in the ventromedial midbrain: Claude's syndrome. J Neurol. 2001;248(12):1087–9.
89. Asakawa H, Yanaka K, Nose T. MRI of Claude's syndrome. Neurology. 2003;61(4):575.
90. Dhanjal T, Walters M, MacMillan N. Claude's syndrome in association with posterior cerebral artery stenosis. Scott Med J. 2003;48(3):91–2.
91. Randhawa S, Donohue MM, Hamilton SR. Concomitant presentation of three rare mesencephalic syndromes: case report. Clin Neurol Neurosurg. 2010;112(8):697–700.
92. Liu GT, Crenner CW, Logigian EL, Charness ME, Samuels MA. Midbrain syndromes of Benedikt, Claude, and Nothnagel: setting the record straight. Neurology. 1992;42(9):1820–2.

Eye Movements and Vestibular Dysfunction: Lesions of Thalamus and Cerebral Cortex

10

The Thalamus

Thalamus is an important relay station between the brainstem and the cerebral cortex. The Fig. 10.1 demonstrates a simplified nuclear arrangement in the cross section of the thalamus. Two thalamic nuclei, intralaminar and ventrolateral, are involved in controlling the eye movements. The intralaminar nuclei, located in the upper wing of the internal medullar lamina, receives input from the frontal, supplementary and parietal eye fields, paramedian pontine reticular formation, superior colliculus, basal ganglia, pretectum, vestibular nuclei, perihypoglossal nuclei and paramedian reticular formation. The projections of the intralaminar nuclei reach the striatum, frontal, supplementary, parietal and cingulate eye fields. The ventrolateral thalamic nuclei receive inputs from the cerebellum and project to the cerebral cortex. Posterolateral thalamus receives input from the vestibular nuclei and deep cerebellar nuclei. Such projections with putatively important role in perception are relayed to the parieto-temporal cortex. Thalamus is one of the common sites for intracranial hemorrhage due to uncontrolled hypertension. Bleeding or structural deficits affecting various parts of the thalamus correlating with specific eye movement and vestibular deficits (Table 10.1).

A. Shaikh, F. Wang, *Eye Movements in the Critical Care Setting*,
https://doi.org/10.1007/978-3-030-70221-2_10

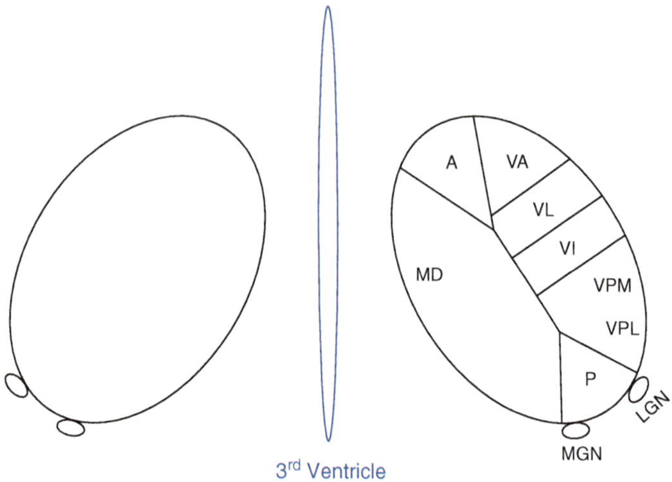

Fig. 10.1 Schematic illustration of axial section through the thalamus. *A* anterior nucleus, *VA* ventroanterior nucleus, *VL* ventrolateral nucleus, *VI* ventrointermedius nucleus, *VPM* ventral postereromedial nucleus, *VPL* ventral posterolateral nucleus, *P* pulvinar nucleus, *MD* mediodorsal nucleus, *MGN* medial geniculate nucleus, *LGN* lateral geniculate nucleus

Table 10.1 Ocular motor dysfunction in thalamic lesions

Central Thalamic	Conjugate gaze deviation away from the side of lesion (wrong way eyes) Sustained downward deviation, sometimes with convergence (peering at the tip of the nose sign) Inward deviation of the eyes (thalamic esotropia) Vertical saccadic palsy when caudal thalamic lesions extend into the rostral mesencephalon Ipsilateral or contralateral tilt of subjective visual vertical
Pulvinar	Difficulty in shifting gaze into contralateral hemifield Hemispatial neglect (especially with acute right-sided lesion)

Central Thalamic Lesions

Central thalamic lesions, typically caused by hemorrhage, leads to contralateral conjugate gaze deviation called "wrong-way eye sign" [1–3]. Such phenomenon is ascribed to the involvement of descending smooth pursuit pathway. Under normal circumstances, smooth pursuit fibers facilitate the eyes to move towards the same side. Lesion of these fibers leads to the deviation of the eyes in the direction away from the lesion [4, 5]. Thalamic hemorrhage can also cause tonic downward deviation of the eyes with convergence miosis, as if the patient is peering at the tip of the nose [1, 6, 7]. Such ocular sign may suggest extension of the hemorrhage or associated edema below mesodiencephalic junction [6]. Cortical descending pathways for divergence pass through the paramedian thalamus and inhibit the contralateral premotor vergence neurons in the midbrain, which projects to the medial rectus subnucleus on the same side [8, 9]. The tonic inward deviation of the eyes is due to the disinhibition of the vergence premotor neurons from the disruption of the cortical descending divergence pathways. Furthermore, the tonic downgaze could also represent compression of the pretectum [10]. Such compression may indicate increased intracranial pressure that can be released by the CSF diversion [11]. Esotropia, an inward deviation of the eyes without downward movements is not uncommon in patients with thalamic lesions as well [8, 12]. The esotropia suggests disruption of the divergence pathways to the medial thalamus. Hemorrhage or structural lesions affecting the posterolateral thalamus can cause subjective false visual perception of the tilt [13–16].

Pulvinar Lesions

Pulvinar nucleus is the largest part in posterior thalamus receiving input from the basal ganglia, parietal and frontal cortices, retina and superior colliculus (Fig. 10.1). Pulvinar neurons have a pivotal role in the visual function, such as suppression of the visual blur during saccades and enhancement of the visual exploration in the contralateral hemispace. Patients with pulvinar lesions have difficulties driving their attention or gaze into the contralesional hemispace. Latter manifest with ipsilateral conjugate gaze deviation or prolonged latency for visually guided saccades to the contralateral hemispace [17, 18]. Such deficit commonly happens on the right-sided lesion. Hence the right pulvinar lesion can mimic right parietal lobe lesion causing hemispatial neglect [19, 20]. Pulvinar is also critical for shifting the visual fixation and target identification [21, 22]. The patients with pulvinar lesions can only perceive and fixate on the ipsilesional target when two visual stimuli appear in each hemifield simultaneously [23]. Patients with pulvinar lesions having inability ignoring the ipsilesional distractors cannot maintain foveation on the target on the contralesional hemifield [24]. Involvement of both pulvinar nuclei can cause photophobia in Wernicke's encephalopathy [25]. In status epilepticus, pulvinar may appear abnormal on MRI but without known clinical consequences [26, 27].

Cerebral Cortex

The cerebral cortex is a common location for ischemic or hemorrhagic strokes that are managed in the critical care units. Although modern imaging modalities are generally the first to reveal the diagnosis, on several occasions ocular signs may provide useful information to monitor the resolution or deterioration of the pathological process (Table 10.2). Acute hemispheric lesions are often associated with conjugate gaze deviation towards the side of the lesion, the "Prevost sign" [28]. There is frequent association of the ipsilateral head rotation along with the eyes [29]. Sustained gaze deviation in patients with right hemispheric lesion are commonly seen when post-Rolandic cortex, subcortical frontal-parietal region, or internal capsule is involved. Visual hemineglect can also cause the gaze preference in patients with right hemispheric lesions [28, 30, 31]. The left hemispheric lesions with persistent gaze deviation are generally large, involving the entire

Table 10.2 Ocular motor dysfunction in cortical lesions

Posterior Occipito-temporal Cortex	Primary visual cortex	Striate cortex is the primary visual cortex Lesion cause contralateral homonymous hemianopia Acutely impaired saccades or pursuit in the blind field Chronic saccade hypometria with increased latency in the blind field.
	MT+ Complex	Human homologues of middle temporal (MT, V5) and medial superior temporal areas (MST) Patients with MT+ complex lesion can experience akinetopsia (loss of motion perception) in contralesional visual field, impairment of ipsiversive pursuit Bilateral MST lesions can cause illusory motion of stationary world during smooth pursuit
Vestibular Cortex (Parieto-insular-vestibular Cortex, PIVC)		Vestibular cortex is in the proximity of the superior temporal gyrus, parietal operculum and posterior insular cortex Lesions lead to the tilted subjective visual vertical to the opposite side Focus of vestibular or tornado epilepsy
Parietal Lobe		Parietal eye filed located in the inferior parietal lobe Acute unilateral parietal lobe lesions cause an ipsilateral horizontal gaze deviation or preference, especially when the lesion is right-sided. Bilateral ptosis can happen and indicates impending herniation. Increased latency in bidirectional saccades (right-sided lesion), increased contraversive saccade latency (left-sided lesion), and impaired ipsiversive smooth pursuit
Frontal Eye Field (FEF)		Middle frontal gyrus with adjacent precentral gyrus Lesions cause ipsilesional eyes and head deviation, diminished or abolished ipsiversive saccades, impaired bidirectional smooth pursuit

(continued)

Table 10.2 (continued)

Supplementary Eye Field (SEF)	Dorsal medial frontal lobe, rostral part of supplementary motor area. Part of network for ocular motor programing. Lesions cause inability to make serially ordered saccades and difficulty making changes in the direction of saccades, also affect predictive ipsilateral smooth pursuit.
Dorsolateral Prefrontal Cortex (DLPC)	Middle frontal gyrus. Part of network for ocular motor programing, inhibition during antisaccades, short-term spatial memory (<25 s) and facilitate predictor saccades. Lesions cause impaired memory-guided saccades and increased antisaccade errors.
Cingulate Eye Field (CEF)	Posterior part of anterior cingulate cortex. Part of network for ocular motor programing, involved in complex behaviors, such as antisaccades and countermanding saccades. Lesions cause increased latency and decreased gain for saccades generation, increased bidirectional errors on antisaccade tasks and memory-guided saccades.

fronto-temporo-parietal region [32]. In most cases, the horizontal gaze deviation results from hemispheric infarct that resolves within a period of 1 week. More persistent gaze deviations suggest pre-existing gaze deviation from the contralateral hemisphere [33]. Conjugate gaze deviations that occur with the supratentorial hemorrhage and persist beyond 72 h predict poor recovery or death [34]. Rarely the cortical hemorrhage can also cause contralesional gaze deviation, “the wrong-way eye sign” [4, 35]. However, most frequently, contralesional gaze deviation in structural cortical lesions suggests seizures. Rarely, extensive bihemispheric lesions as seen in bilateral infarctions in the vascular distribution of the middle cerebral artery cause complete volitional ophthalmoplegia. This phenomenon is also called anterior opercular syndrome or Foix-Chavany-Marie syndrome, which features preserved vestibular eye movements secondary to injured subcortical white matter leading to deafferentation of superior colliculus and brainstem structures [36–38].

Large hemispheric lesions can present with deficits in the saccades towards the contralesional hemisphere, ipsilateral smooth pursuits, optokinetic response, and vestibulo-ocular reflex (VOR) cancellation [39]. Horizontal nystagmus with quick-phase beating towards the lesioned hemisphere can be present and it suggests unopposed pursuit or vestibular drive drifting the eyes towards to contralateral intact hemisphere [40, 41].

Hemispheric lesions increase saccade latency in both ipsilesional and contralesional sides. The prolongation in the latency can be multifactorial, due to, hemianopia, visual attention deficit, or impaired motor planning. Saccadic accuracy can be impaired as well with contralesionally directed saccades being hypometric. Smaller frontal and parietal lesions can cause increased directional errors while making antisaccades, and inappropriate saccades during memory-guided saccade tasks [42]. The above deficits in acute settings may suggest recovery from the acute lesions.

The vertical saccades may have uncalled-for horizontal component making the trajectory curve towards the contralateral hemisphere [43]. The deficits are especially profound with non-dominant hemispheric lesion [44]. Commonly seen with parieto-temporal deficits, forced closure of the eyelids associates with contralateral "spastic" conjugate gaze deviation [45–47]. Unlike ipsipulsion, such phenomenology is only present with eye closure.

Posterior Occipital-Temporal Cortex

Occipital lobe lesions affecting the striate cortex (V1) not only cause contralateral homonymous hemianopia but also ocular motor deficits. Figure 10.2 demonstrates a left primary visual cortex lesion. In the acute phase the patients may not be able to generate saccades or pursuit to the blind hemifield. Later, saccades in

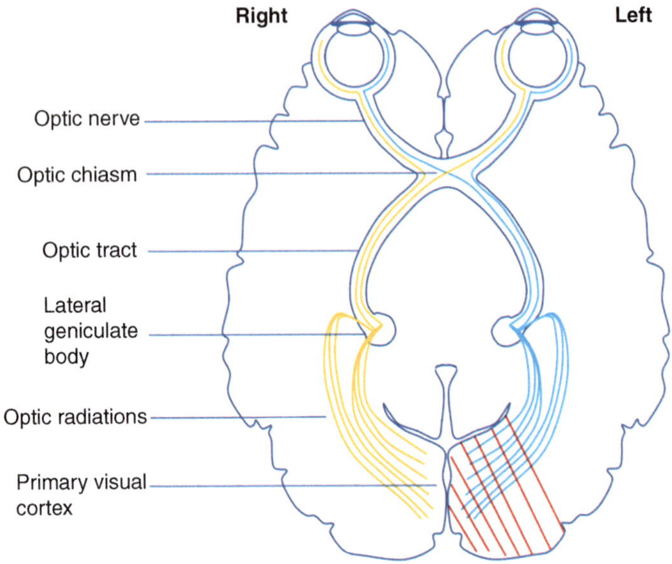

Fig. 10.2 Schematic illustration of the visual pathway and the lesion in the left primary visual cortex (V1). The lesion causes contralateral homonymous hemianopia, but the eye movement abnormality can be present. In the acute phase, the patient may not be able to generate voluntary movements to the stimuli on the right side. Subsequently, the saccades become hypometric with increased latency to the right side

the hemianopic field are hypometric with increased latency [48, 49]. Similar patterns were also noted in response to voice stimuli in some patients, implying striate cortex also participates in motor planning to some extent [50]. Patients with hemianopia frequently develop different compensatory strategies to improve eye movement accuracy, unless hemineglect coexists [48, 51]. These strategies include but are not limited to the series of small searching saccades, overshooting saccades to bring the target into the intact visual field, and prediction with memory-guided saccades. Furthermore, the presence of these strategies can be used to detect hemineglect [52]. Similarly, combined head and eye movements can have increased latency of head movements and development of compensatory strategies while looking into the hemianopic side [48, 53].

Smooth pursuit remains relatively intact with unilateral V1 lesions if the stimulus is presented to the intact visual field; optokinetic response in the intact hemifield is also normal [54]. However, the motion detection in the blind hemifield is impaired [55]. Functional imaging studies suggested that the secondary visual areas at occipital-temporal cortex, Brodmann areas 39 and 40, are activated by moving stimuli via the activation of either direct extrastriatal visual pathways or interhemispheric callosal connections between both MT+ complexes [56].

Patients with cortical blindness caused by bilateral occipital lesions, the Anton syndrome, often do not recognize their visual loss but instead confabulate of what they see. Akinetopsia, the impaired visual motion perception, is present in patients with lesions affecting unilateral MT+ complex [57–59]. Such patients may also have retinotopic deficits of smooth pursuit and saccadic interruption [60, 61]. The patients with more diffuse cerebral lesions may present with impaired or complete loss of motion perception suggesting dispersed motion perception network [58, 62]. Unilateral lesion involving the adjacent MT+ complex produces tracking deficits showing ipsilateral pursuit impairment and difficulty in perceiving the motion in the contralateral visual field [60, 61, 63–66]. Bilateral medial superior temporal cortex lesions cause illusory motion of the stationary world during smooth pursuit; the patients are unable to distinguish whether the world is truly moving or not [67].

Vestibular Cortex (Parieto-Insular-Vestibular Cortex, PIVC)

Vestibular cortex locates at the junction of superior temporal gyrus, parietal operculum and posterior insular cortex, and is instrumental for the perception of self-motion and spatial orientation. The lesion at this location causes the subjective visual vertical tilting to contralateral side, abolishes the sense of self-rotation and spatial navigation, leads to bodily perception abnormalities, and impairs memory-guided saccades [68–72]. Rarely an acute infarct involving right vestibular cortex can present with acute vestibular syndrome, but the lesion confined to the insular cortex typically does not cause vestibular deficits [73, 74]. Temporal lobe seizure can present with a wide range of vestibular sensations from nonspecific dizziness to a sensation of rotation, vestibular or "tornado" epilepsy [75–78].

Parietal Lobe

Acute unilateral parietal lobe lesions often cause an ipsilateral gaze preference and bilateral ptosis; the constellation often indicate impending herniation [79]. Ocular motor deficits in parietal lobe lesions can be partly explained by hemineglect. Latency of visually guided saccades to either direction may be increased in right-sided lesions especially when the inferior parietal sulcus, the parietal eye field, is affected [80]. Left parietal lesion, however, only affects rightward saccades [81].

Individuals with hemispatial neglect have difficulties attending visual information in the neglected hemispace [82]. Moreover, searching behaviors within neglected hemispace demonstrate a combination of spatial bias and loss of working memory [83, 84]. During visual search, patients' eyes return too frequently to the fixation point that they have previously visited. In patients with hemispatial neglect, saccadic reaction time is influenced by the position of the eyes in the orbit, with reaction time being greater when the eyes are on the lesion side [85]. There is also some evidence showing that repetitive contralesional smooth-pursuit "training" promotes recovery from the neglect [86].

Asymmetry of smooth pursuit and optokinetic reflex were also traditionally attributed to the parietal lobe lesions. However, functional imaging studies indicated that the involvement of the secondary visual areas are more concerned with motion perception [65]. Lesions involving these regions contribute to the impaired smooth tracking [65]. In patients with injury involving inferior parietal cortex or parieto-frontal connections, they tend to have more trouble with pursuit while tracking a target moving across structured background versus dark background [87]. This finding also supports the relatively spared full-filed optokinetic responses in patients with parietal lesions, since optokinetic reflexes requires less attention [88]. Bilateral parietal lesions can cause optic ataxia, ocular motor apraxia and simultanagnosia, i.e., Balint's syndrome as elaborated in the subsequent section [89].

Acquired Ocular Motor Apraxia

Acute bilateral frontal, fronto-parietal or parietal lobe lesions can produce acquired ocular motor apraxia [90–94]. Because frontal and parietal eye fields are within the watershed zone of the major intracranial vessels, they are susceptible to vascular insults. Acquired ocular motor apraxia is best characterized by loss of volitional control of any eye movements, with preservation of the reflexive eye movements, such as VOR (both slow and quick phases). Because of the right parietal lobe involvement, left-sided hemineglect can be present with ocular motor apraxia. Patients may have difficulties in initiating volitional saccades to command, however could often shift gaze by making combined head-eye movements, usually with blinking. The reflexive quick-phase of the eye movements can be present during head impulse test or optokinetic stimuli presentation. Smooth pursuit is also impaired [95]. The constellation of symptoms likely reflects a disruption of both frontal eye field and parietal eye field pathways, hence, the structures in the final common pathway for the eye movements, such as superior colliculus, cerebellum and brainstem structures, are deprived of cortical inputs. The Fig. 10.3 demonstrates the theoretical connections for eye movements pathway. This theory was proven by using the animal models with experimental ablations in either bilateral frontal eye fields and superior colliculus or frontal and parietal eye fields [96, 97]. The fact that head-eye movements could help shift gaze directions could imply an independent process [98, 99]. On the other hand, blinking helps promote saccade generation by inhibiting omnipause neurons, and thus allowing excitatory burst neurons to generate saccades [100].

Balint's syndrome consists of ocular motor apraxia, optic ataxia (inaccurate finger pointing) and simultanagnosia (disturbance of visual attention) [57, 90, 101–106]. Various disorders affecting bilateral fronto-parietal cortices might cause Balint's syndrome and its variants, including watershed and embolic infarcts, neoplastic process, pre-eclampsia/eclampsia, demyelin-

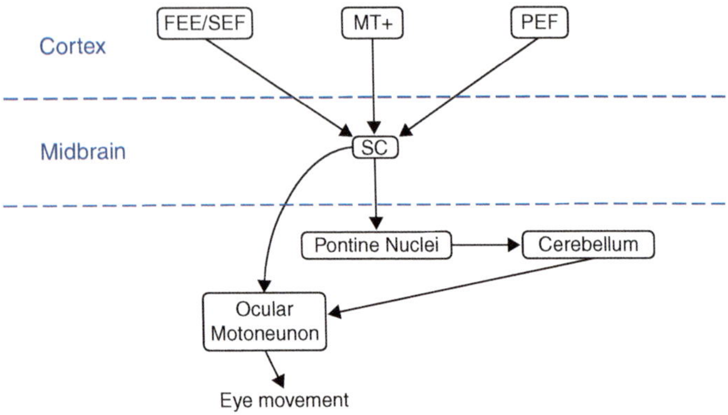

Fig. 10.3 Simplified scheme of connections between each cortical eye field and final common pathway. Disconnection between parietal lobe or frontal lobe and brainstem on both sides can lead to acquired ocular motor apraxia

ation, degenerative and autoimmune disorders, and non-convulsive status epilepticus [107–120]. If it was caused by bilateral parieto-occipital lesions, voluntary saccades can be more easily generated toward visual stimuli because such process is mainly attributed to frontal eye field [89]. Deficits in saccades can manifest as increased latency, dysmetria, and inability to perform visual search [121–123].

Frontal Lobe

There are at least four areas within frontal lobe that are pertinent to the control of eye movements; the frontal eye field (FEF), supplementary eye field (SEF), dorsolateral prefrontal cortex (DLPC), and cingulate gyrus (CEF).

Frontal Eye Field (FEF)

Frontal eye field is located in the middle frontal gyrus and adjacent precentral gyrus, between Brodmann areas 4, 6 and 8. Acute lesions involving FEF cause ipsilateral gaze and head deviation which resolves with time [29, 124]. In addition to gaze deviation, the FEF lesions also lead to visual fixation abnormalities due to excessive spontaneous ipsiversive saccades secondary to the imbalance of FEF inputs [43]. In animal experiments, inactivation of FEF also causes increased latency, dysmetria and decreased velocity of the ipsiversive saccades [125]. Contralateral gaze deviation had also been described in patients with acute frontal hemorrhage and frontoparietal lesions [4, 35, 126]. Acute bifrontal lesions cause ocular motor apraxia.

FEF lesions also affect smooth pursuit [44, 65, 127–130]. Unilateral FEF lesion causes bilateral horizontal pursuit abnormalities, with more severe impairment in the ipsilesional pursuit. The FEF lesions affect both the initiation as well as the maintenance of pursuit. The FEF also houses the neurons ensuring visual fixation, hence its lesion can lead to frequent unwanted saccades interrupting the fixation [131]. The FEF also facilitates vergence and three-dimensional tracking [132, 133]. The frontal lobe epilepsy can sometimes lead to disconjugate gaze deviation [134].

Supplementary Eye Field (SEF)

SEF is in the dorsal medial frontal lobe, in the rostral part of the supplementary motor area (Brodmann area 6). It is the part of the neural network that includes presupplementary cortex, cingulate cortex and hippocampus that is responsible for motor programming and learned behaviors. Thus, SEF lesions cause loss of abilities to make sequenced saccades, especially with left-sided lesion [135–137]. Another deficit commonly associated with SEF injury is difficulty in modifying the direction of saccades from either a previous intention or the behavioral goal [138]. The SEF lesions can also affect predictive, ipsiversive smooth pursuit [44, 65].

Dorsolateral Prefrontal Cortex (DLPC)

DLPC also locates in the middle frontal gyrus, and has an important role in the ocular motor programming process, preparing saccades by suppressing unwanted saccades, maintaining short-term spatial memory and facilitating anticipatory saccades [139]. The patients with right DLPC lesions have defective memory-guided saccades and increased numbers of errors on antisaccade task

[140, 141]. Increased distractibility and increased errors on anti-saccade task can be observed as a result of disruption of direct prefrontotectal tract [142–144]. DLPC lesions are also associated with bidirectional pursuit deficits [44].

Cingulate Eye Field (CEF)

CEF is near the posterior aspect of the anterior cingulate cortex. It is involved in the performance of complex behaviors, such as antisaccades and countermanding saccades [145–152]. Small infarcts in the right CEF lead to increased latency and decreased gain of saccades [145]. The patient also makes increased numbers of bidirectional errors on antisaccade and memory-guided saccade tasks [153].

Summary

In this chapter, we reviewed the two important parts of brain structures involving in the higher chains of command for eye movements – thalamus and cortex. Thalamus is the relay station between brainstem and cortex. Grossly, two separate divisions of thalamus are concerned with eye movements – central thalamic nucleus and pulvinar nucleus. Lesions of central thalamic nucleus could present with a wide variety of clinical signs – wrong way eyes, peering at the tip of the nose, thalamic esotropia and tilt of subjective vertical. On the other hand, pulvinar injury typically causes difficulty with attention and neglect. There are multiple regions coordinating and processing all the eye movements – frontal eye field (FEF), supplementary eye field (SEF), dorsolateral prefrontal cortex (DLPC), cingulate eye field (CEF), parietal eye field (PEF), vestibular cortex, MT+ complex and primary visual cortex. Out of these areas, FEF is concerned with saccades function. SEF, DLPC and CEF form a complex network for ocular motor programming and planning. PEF mainly contributes to the pursuit function. Vestibular cortex and MT+ help perceive the depth and velocity of images. And primary visual cortex is the location for visual perception.

References

1. Fisher CM. The pathologic and clinical aspects of thalamic hemorrhage. Trans Am Neurol Assoc. 1959;84:56–9.
2. Keane JR. Contralateral gaze deviation with supratentorial hemorrhage. Arch Neurol. 1975;32(2):119–22.
3. Tijssen CC. Contralateral conjugate eye deviation in acute supratentorial lesions. Stroke. 1994;25(7):1516–9.
4. Sharpe JA, Bondar RL, Fletcher WA. Contralateral gaze deviation after frontal lobe haemorrhage. J Neurol Neurosurg Psychiatry. 1985;48(1):86–8.
5. Tanaka M. Involvement of the central thalamus in the control of smooth pursuit eye movements. J Neurosci. 2005;25(25):5866–76.
6. Choi KD, Jung DS, Kim JS. Specificity of "peering at the tip of the nose" for a diagnosis of thalamic hemorrhage. Arch Neurol. 2004;61(3):417–22.
7. Ahmad KE, Kumar KR. "Peering at the tip of the nose" as a sign of thalamic haemorrhage. Neuroophthalmology. 2014;38(1):21–3.
8. Gomez CR, Gomez SM, Selhorst JB. Acute thalamic esotropia. Neurology. 1988;38(11):1759–62.
9. Wiest G, Mallek R, Baumgartner C. Selective loss of vergence control secondary to bilateral paramedian thalamic infarction. Neurology. 2000;54(10):1997–9.
10. Siatkowski RM, Schatz NJ, Sellitti TP, Galetta SL, Glaser JS. Do thalamic lesions really cause vertical gaze palsies? J Clin Neuroophthalmol. 1993;13(3):190–3.
11. Waga S, Okada M, Yamamoto Y. Reversibility of Parinaud syndrome in thalamic hemorrhage. Neurology. 1979;29(3):407–9.
12. Hertle RW, Bienfang DC. Oculographic analysis of acute esotropia secondary to a thalamic hemorrhage. J Clin Neuroophthalmol. 1990;10(1):21–6.
13. Dieterich M, Brandt T. Thalamic infarctions: differential effects on vestibular function in the roll plane (35 patients). Neurology. 1993;43(9):1732–40.
14. Baier B, Vogt T, Rohde F, Cuvenhaus H, Conrad J, Dieterich M. Deep brain stimulation of the nucleus ventralis intermedius: a thalamic site of graviceptive modulation. Brain Struct Funct. 2017;222(1):645–50.
15. Baier B, Conrad J, Stephan T, Kirsch V, Vogt T, Wilting J, et al. Vestibular thalamus: two distinct graviceptive pathways. Neurology. 2016;86(2):134–40.
16. Glasauer S, Dieterich M, Brandt T. Neuronal network-based mathematical modeling of perceived verticality in acute unilateral vestibular lesions: from nerve to thalamus and cortex. J Neurol. 2018;265(Suppl 1):101–12.

17. Rafal R, McGrath M, Machado L, Hindle J. Effects of lesions of the human posterior thalamus on ocular fixation during voluntary and visually triggered saccades. J Neurol Neurosurg Psychiatry. 2004;75(11):1602–6.
18. Ogren MP, Mateer CA, Wyler AR. Alterations in visually related eye movements following left pulvinar damage in man. Neuropsychologia. 1984;22(2):187–96.
19. Karnath HO, Himmelbach M, Rorden C. The subcortical anatomy of human spatial neglect: putamen, caudate nucleus and pulvinar. Brain. 2002;125(Pt 2):350–60.
20. Arend I, Rafal R, Ward R. Spatial and temporal deficits are regionally dissociable in patients with pulvinar lesions. Brain. 2008;131(Pt 8):2140–52.
21. Wilke M, Turchi J, Smith K, Mishkin M, Leopold DA. Pulvinar inactivation disrupts selection of movement plans. J Neurosci. 2010;30(25):8650–9.
22. Strumpf H, Mangun GR, Boehler CN, Stoppel C, Schoenfeld MA, Heinze HJ, et al. The role of the pulvinar in distractor processing and visual search. Hum Brain Mapp. 2013;34(5):1115–32.
23. Arend I, Machado L, Ward R, McGrath M, Ro T, Rafal RD. The role of the human pulvinar in visual attention and action: evidence from temporal-order judgment, saccade decision, and antisaccade tasks. Prog Brain Res. 2008;171:475–83.
24. Van der Stigchel S, Arend I, van Koningsbruggen MG, Rafal RD. Oculomotor integration in patients with a pulvinar lesion. Neuropsychologia. 2010;48(12):3497–504.
25. Rosini F, Cerase A, Pretegiani E, Lucii G, Federighi P, Federico A, et al. Photophobia and bilateral pulvinar involvement in non-alcoholic Wernicke's encephalopathy. Neurol Sci. 2013;34(10):1867–9.
26. Ohe Y, Hayashi T, Deguchi I, Fukuoka T, Horiuchi Y, Maruyama H, et al. MRI abnormality of the pulvinar in patients with status epilepticus. J Neuroradiol. 2014;41(4):220–6.
27. Nakae Y, Kudo Y, Yamamoto R, Dobashi Y, Kawabata Y, Ikeda S, et al. Relationship between cortex and pulvinar abnormalities on diffusion-weighted imaging in status epilepticus. J Neurol. 2016;263(1):127–32.
28. Singer OC, Humpich MC, Laufs H, Lanfermann H, Steinmetz H, Neumann-Haefelin T. Conjugate eye deviation in acute stroke: incidence, hemispheric asymmetry, and lesion pattern. Stroke. 2006;37(11):2726–32.
29. Tanaka H, Arai M, Kubo J, Hirata K. Conjugate eye deviation with head version due to a cortical infarction of the frontal eye field. Stroke. 2002;33(2):642–3.
30. Fruhmann Berger M, Pross RD, Ilg U, Karnath HO. Deviation of eyes and head in acute cerebral stroke. BMC Neurol. 2006;6:23.

31. Fruhmann Berger M, Johannsen L, Karnath HO. Time course of eye and head deviation in spatial neglect. Neuropsychology. 2008;22(6):697–702.
32. Tijssen CC, van Gisbergen JA, Schulte BP. Conjugate eye deviation: side, site, and size of the hemispheric lesion. Neurology. 1991;41(6):846–50.
33. Steiner I, Melamed E. Conjugate eye deviation after acute hemispheric stroke: delayed recovery after previous contralateral frontal lobe damage. Ann Neurol. 1984;16(4):509–11.
34. Sato S, Koga M, Yamagami H, Okuda S, Okada Y, Kimura K, et al. Conjugate eye deviation in acute intracerebral hemorrhage: stroke acute management with urgent risk-factor assessment and improvement--ICH (SAMURAI-ICH) study. Stroke. 2012;43(11):2898–903.
35. Pessin MS, Adelman LS, Prager RJ, Lathi ES, Lange DJ. "Wrong-way eyes" in supratentorial hemorrhage. Ann Neurol. 1981;9(1):79–81.
36. Foix C. Diplégie facio-linguo-masticatrice d'origine cortico sous-corticale sans paralysie des membres (contribution à l'étude de la localisation des centres de la face et du membre superieur). Rev Neurol. 1926;33:214–9.
37. Weller M. Anterior opercular cortex lesions cause dissociated lower cranial nerve palsies and anarthria but no aphasia: Foix-Chavany-Marie syndrome and "automatic voluntary dissociation" revisited. J Neurol. 1993;240(4):199–208.
38. Jadhav AP, Zenonos G, Pless M, Jovin TG, Wechsler L. A variant of the anterior opercular syndrome with supranuclear gaze palsy. JAMA Neurol. 2013;70(6):800–1.
39. Morrow MJ. Craniotopic defects of smooth pursuit and saccadic eye movement. Neurology. 1996;46(2):514–21.
40. Tusa RJ, Zee DS, Herdman SJ. Effect of unilateral cerebral cortical lesions on ocular motor behavior in monkeys: saccades and quick phases. J Neurophysiol. 1986;56(6):1590–625.
41. Sharpe JA, Lo AW, Rabinovitch HE. Control of the saccadic and smooth pursuit systems after cerebral hemidecortication. Brain. 1979;102(2):387–403.
42. Dong W, Yan B, Johnson BP, Millist L, Davis S, Fielding J, et al. Ischaemic stroke: the ocular motor system as a sensitive marker for motor and cognitive recovery. J Neurol Neurosurg Psychiatry. 2013;84(3):337–41.
43. Dias EC, Segraves MA. Muscimol-induced inactivation of monkey frontal eye field: effects on visually and memory-guided saccades. J Neurophysiol. 1999;81(5):2191–214.
44. Lekwuwa GU, Barnes GR. Cerebral control of eye movements. I. The relationship between cerebral lesion sites and smooth pursuit deficits. Brain. 1996;119(Pt 2):473–90.

45. Cogan DG. Neurologic significance of lateral conjugate deviation of the eyes on forced closure of the lids. Arch Ophthalmol. 1948;39(1):37–42.
46. Smith JL, Gay AJ, Cogan DG. The spasticity of conjugate gaze phenomenon. Arch Ophthalmol. 1959;62:694–6.
47. Sullivan HC, Kaminski HJ, Maas EF, Weissman JD, Leigh RJ. Lateral deviation of the eyes on forced lid closure in patients with cerebral lesions. Arch Neurol. 1991;48(3):310–1.
48. Fayel A, Chokron S, Cavezian C, Vergilino-Perez D, Lemoine C, Dore-Mazars K. Characteristics of contralesional and ipsilesional saccades in hemianopic patients. Exp Brain Res. 2014;232(3):903–17.
49. Reinhard JI, Damm I, Ivanov IV, Trauzettel-Klosinski S. Eye movements during saccadic and fixation tasks in patients with homonymous hemianopia. J Neuroophthalmol. 2014;34(4):354–61.
50. Traccis S, Puliga MV, Ruiu MC, Marras MA, Rosati G. Unilateral occipital lesion causing hemianopia affects the acoustic saccadic programming. Neurology. 1991;41(10):1633–8.
51. Meienberg O, Zangemeister WH, Rosenberg M, Hoyt WF, Stark L. Saccadic eye movement strategies in patients with homonymous hemianopia. Ann Neurol. 1981;9(6):537–44.
52. Meienberg O. Clinical examination of saccadic eye movements in hemianopia. Neurology. 1983;33(10):1311–5.
53. Zangemeister WH, Meienberg O, Stark L, Hoyt WF. Eye-head coordination in homonymous hemianopia. J Neurol. 1982;226(4):243–54.
54. Segraves MA, Goldberg ME, Deng SY, Bruce CJ, Ungerleider LG, Mishkin M. The role of striate cortex in the guidance of eye movements in the monkey. J Neurosci. 1987;7(10):3040–58.
55. Barton JJ, Sharpe JA. Motion direction discrimination in blind hemifields. Ann Neurol. 1997;41(2):255–64.
56. Brandt T, Bucher SF, Seelos KC, Dieterich M. Bilateral functional MRI activation of the basal ganglia and middle temporal/medial superior temporal motion-sensitive areas: optokinetic stimulation in homonymous hemianopia. Arch Neurol. 1998;55(8):1126–31.
57. Barton JJ. Disorders of higher visual processing. Handb Clin Neurol. 2011;102:223–61.
58. Cooper SA, Joshi AC, Seenan PJ, Hadley DM, Muir KW, Leigh RJ, et al. Akinetopsia: acute presentation and evidence for persisting defects in motion vision. J Neurol Neurosurg Psychiatry. 2012;83(2):229–30.
59. Shipp S, de Jong BM, Zihl J, Frackowiak RS, Zeki S. The brain activity related to residual motion vision in a patient with bilateral lesions of V5. Brain. 1994;117(Pt 5):1023–38.
60. Thurston SE, Leigh RJ, Crawford T, Thompson A, Kennard C. Two distinct deficits of visual tracking caused by unilateral lesions of cerebral cortex in humans. Ann Neurol. 1988;23(3):266–73.
61. Dursteler MR, Wurtz RH. Pursuit and optokinetic deficits following chemical lesions of cortical areas MT and MST. J Neurophysiol. 1988;60(3):940–65.

62. Gilaie-Dotan S, Saygin AP, Lorenzi LJ, Egan R, Rees G, Behrmann M. The role of human ventral visual cortex in motion perception. Brain. 2013;136(Pt 9):2784–98.
63. Barton JJ, Sharpe JA, Raymond JE. Retinotopic and directional defects in motion discrimination in humans with cerebral lesions. Ann Neurol. 1995;37(5):665–75.
64. Barton JJ, Sharpe JA, Raymond JE. Directional defects in pursuit and motion perception in humans with unilateral cerebral lesions. Brain. 1996;119(Pt 5):1535–50.
65. Heide W, Kurzidim K, Kompf D. Deficits of smooth pursuit eye movements after frontal and parietal lesions. Brain. 1996;119(Pt 6):1951–69.
66. Morrow MJ, Sharpe JA. Retinotopic and directional deficits of smooth pursuit initiation after posterior cerebral hemispheric lesions. Neurology. 1993;43(3 Pt 1):595–603.
67. Haarmeier T, Thier P, Repnow M, Petersen D. False perception of motion in a patient who cannot compensate for eye movements. Nature. 1997;389(6653):849–52.
68. Taube JS. The head direction signal: origins and sensory-motor integration. Annu Rev Neurosci. 2007;30:181–207.
69. Dieterich M, Brandt T. Perception of verticality and vestibular disorders of balance and falls. Front Neurol. 2019;10:172.
70. Straube A, Brandt T. Importance of the visual and vestibular cortex for self-motion perception in man (circularvection). Hum Neurobiol. 1987;6(3):211–8.
71. Israel I, Rivaud S, Gaymard B, Berthoz A, Pierrot-Deseilligny C. Cortical control of vestibular-guided saccades in man. Brain. 1995;118(Pt 5):1169–83.
72. Lopez C. A neuroscientific account of how vestibular disorders impair bodily self-consciousness. Front Integr Neurosci. 2013;7:91.
73. von Brevern M, Sussmilch S, Zeise D. Acute vertigo due to hemispheric stroke: a case report and comprehensive review of the literature. J Neurol Sci. 2014;339(1–2):153–6.
74. Baier B, Conrad J, Zu Eulenburg P, Best C, Muller-Forell W, Birklein F, et al. Insular strokes cause no vestibular deficits. Stroke. 2013;44(9):2604–6.
75. Nielsen JM. Tornado epilepsy simulating Meniere's syndrome: report of 4 cases. Neurology. 1959;9:794–6.
76. Ahmed I. Epilepsia tornado. J Kans Med Soc. 1980;81(10):466–7.
77. Erbayat Altay E, Serdaroglu A, Gucuyener K, Bilir E, Karabacak NI, Thio LL. Rotational vestibular epilepsy from the temporo-parieto-occipital junction. Neurology. 2005;65(10):1675–6.
78. Hewett R, Bartolomei F. Epilepsy and the cortical vestibular system: tales of dizziness and recent concepts. Front Integr Neurosci. 2013;7:73.
79. Averbuch-Heller L, Leigh RJ, Mermelstein V, Zagalsky L, Streifler JY. Ptosis in patients with hemispheric strokes. Neurology. 2002;58(4):620–4.

80. Ptak R, Muri RM. The parietal cortex and saccade planning: lessons from human lesion studies. Front Hum Neurosci. 2013;7:254.
81. Pierrot-Deseilligny C, Rivaud S, Gaymard B, Agid Y. Cortical control of reflexive visually-guided saccades. Brain. 1991;114(Pt 3):1473–85.
82. Kennard C. Scanpaths: the path to understanding abnormal cognitive processing in neurological disease. Ann N Y Acad Sci. 2002;956:242–9.
83. Husain M, Mannan S, Hodgson T, Wojciulik E, Driver J, Kennard C. Impaired spatial working memory across saccades contributes to abnormal search in parietal neglect. Brain. 2001;124(Pt 5):941–52.
84. van Koningsbruggen MG, Gabay S, Sapir A, Henik A, Rafal RD. Hemispheric asymmetry in the remapping and maintenance of visual saliency maps: a TMS study. J Cogn Neurosci. 2010;22(8): 1730–8.
85. Behrmann M, Ghiselli-Crippa T, Sweeney JA, Di Matteo I, Kass R. Mechanisms underlying spatial representation revealed through studies of hemispatial neglect. J Cogn Neurosci. 2002;14(2):272–90.
86. Kerkhoff G, Reinhart S, Ziegler W, Artinger F, Marquardt C, Keller I. Smooth pursuit eye movement training promotes recovery from auditory and visual neglect: a randomized controlled study. Neurorehabil Neural Repair. 2013;27(9):789–98.
87. Lawden MC, Bagelmann H, Crawford TJ, Matthews TD, Kennard C. An effect of structured backgrounds on smooth pursuit eye movements in patients with cerebral lesions. Brain. 1995;118(Pt 1):37–48.
88. Baloh RW, Yee RD, Honrubia V. Optokinetic nystagmus and parietal lobe lesions. Ann Neurol. 1980;7(3):269–76.
89. Pierrot-Deseilligny C, Gray F, Brunet P. Infarcts of both inferior parietal lobules with impairment of visually guided eye movements, peripheral visual inattention and optic ataxia. Brain. 1986;109(Pt 1):81–97.
90. Pierrot-Deseilligny C, Gautier JC, Loron P. Acquired ocular motor apraxia due to bilateral frontoparietal infarcts. Ann Neurol. 1988;23(2):199–202.
91. Dehaene I, Lammens M. Paralysis of saccades and pursuit: clinicopathologic study. Neurology. 1991;41(3):414–5.
92. Genc BO, Genc E, Acik L, Ilhan S, Paksoy Y. Acquired ocular motor apraxia from bilateral frontoparietal infarcts associated with Takayasu arteritis. J Neurol Neurosurg Psychiatry. 2004;75(11):1651–2.
93. Rambold H, Moser A, Zurowski B, Gbadamosi J, Kompf D, Sprenger A, et al. Saccade initiation in ocular motor apraxia. J Neurol. 2006;253(7):950–2.
94. Chen JJ, Thurtell MJ. Neurological picture. Acquired ocular motor apraxia due to bifrontal haemorrhages. J Neurol Neurosurg Psychiatry. 2012;83(11):1117–8.
95. Leigh RJ, Tusa RJ. Disturbance of smooth pursuit caused by infarction of occipitoparietal cortex. Ann Neurol. 1985;17(2):185–7.

96. Schiller PH, True SD, Conway JL. Deficits in eye movements following frontal eye-field and superior colliculus ablations. J Neurophysiol. 1980;44(6):1175–89.
97. Lynch JC. Saccade initiation and latency deficits after combined lesions of the frontal and posterior eye fields in monkeys. J Neurophysiol. 1992;68(5):1913–6.
98. Corneil BD, Olivier E, Munoz DP. Visual responses on neck muscles reveal selective gating that prevents express saccades. Neuron. 2004;42(5):831–41.
99. Corneil BD, Elsley JK. Countermanding eye-head gaze shifts in humans: marching orders are delivered to the head first. J Neurophysiol. 2005;94(1):883–95.
100. Mays LE, Morrisse DW. Electrical stimulation of the pontine omnipause area inhibits eye blink. J Am Optom Assoc. 1995;66(7):419–22.
101. Holmes G. Disturbances of visual orientation. Br J Ophthalmol. 1918;2(9):449–68.
102. Cogan DG. Ophthalmic manifestations of bilateral non-occipital cerebral lesions. Br J Ophthalmol. 1965;49:281–97.
103. Husain M, Stein J. Rezso Balint and his most celebrated case. Arch Neurol. 1988;45(1):89–93.
104. Johnston JL, Sharpe JA, Morrow MJ. Spasm of fixation: a quantitative study. J Neurol Sci. 1992;107(2):166–71.
105. Balslev D, Odoj B, Rennig J, Karnath HO. Abnormal center-periphery gradient in spatial attention in simultanagnosia. J Cogn Neurosci. 2014;26(12):2778–88.
106. Andersen RA, Andersen KN, Hwang EJ, Hauschild M. Optic ataxia: from Balint's syndrome to the parietal reach region. Neuron. 2014;81(5):967–83.
107. Berti A, Papagno C, Vallar G. Balint syndrome: a case of simultanagnosia. Ital J Neurol Sci. 1986;7(2):261–4.
108. Mendez MF, Turner J, Gilmore GC, Remler B, Tomsak RL. Balint's syndrome in Alzheimer's disease: visuospatial functions. Int J Neurosci. 1990;54(3–4):339–46.
109. Mendez MF, Cherrier MM. The evolution of alexia and simultanagnosia in posterior cortical atrophy. Neuropsychiatry Neuropsychol Behav Neurol. 1998;11(2):76–82.
110. Ances BM, Ellenbogen JM, Herman ST, Jacobs D, Liebeskind DS, Chatterjee A, et al. Balint syndrome due to Creutzfeldt-Jakob disease. Neurology. 2004;63(2):395.
111. Areza-Fegyveres R, Caramelli P, Porto CS, Ono CR, Buchpiguel CA, Nitrini R. The syndrome of progressive posterior cortical dysfunction: a multiple case study and review. Dement Neuropsychol. 2007;1(3):311–9.
112. Mejia NI, Park S, Ning M, Buonanno FS. Pearls and Oy-sters: reversible iatrogenic Balint syndrome. Neurology. 2008;70(24):e97–8.

113. Kumar S, Abhayambika A, Sundaram AN, Sharpe JA. Posterior reversible encephalopathy syndrome presenting as Balint syndrome. J Neuroophthalmol. 2011;31(3):224–7.
114. Ristic AJ, Marjanovic I, Brajkovic L, Wolgamuth BR, Odalovic S, Lavrnic S, et al. Balint-like syndrome as an unusual representation of non-convulsive status epilepticus. Epileptic Disord. 2012;14(1):80–4.
115. Rajagopal R, Bateman R, Van Stavern GP. Visual involvement in corticobasal syndrome. J Neuroophthalmol. 2012;32(4):338–40.
116. Chechlacz M, Humphreys GW. The enigma of Balint's syndrome: neural substrates and cognitive deficits. Front Hum Neurosci. 2014;8:123.
117. Beh SC, Muthusamy B, Calabresi P, Hart J, Zee D, Patel V, et al. Hiding in plain sight: a closer look at posterior cortical atrophy. Pract Neurol. 2015;15(1):5–13.
118. Sakurai Y, Nakashima Y. Progressive Balint's syndrome in a patient demonstrating dementia with lewy bodies. Intern Med. 2017;56(11):1421–4.
119. Godel M, Ptak R, Schnider A, Nicastro N. Balint syndrome caused by bilateral medial occipital infarcts. Neurol Sci. 2018;39(10):1813–4.
120. Metzger A, Pisella L, Vighetto A, Joubert B, Honnorat J, Tilikete C, et al. Balint syndrome in anti-NMDA receptor encephalitis. Neurol Neuroimmunol Neuroinflamm. 2019;6(1):e532.
121. Zihl J, Hebel N. Patterns of oculomotor scanning in patients with unilateral posterior parietal or frontal lobe damage. Neuropsychologia. 1997;35(6):893–906.
122. Behrmann M, Watt S, Black SE, Barton JJ. Impaired visual search in patients with unilateral neglect: an oculographic analysis. Neuropsychologia. 1997;35(11):1445–58.
123. Ptak R, Fellrath J. Exploring the world with Balint syndrome: biased bottom-up guidance of gaze by local saliency differences. Exp Brain Res. 2014;232(4):1233–40.
124. Daroff R, Hoyt W. Supranuclear disorders of ocular control systems in man. In: The control of eye movements. New York: Academic Press; 1971. p. 175–235.
125. Peel TR, Johnston K, Lomber SG, Corneil BD. Bilateral saccadic deficits following large and reversible inactivation of unilateral frontal eye field. J Neurophysiol. 2014;111(2):415–33.
126. Park JW, Choi JY, Jung JM, Kwon DY, Park MH, Kim JS. Contralesional spasticity of conjugate gaze in striatocapsular infarction. Can J Neurol Sci. 2014;41(2):270–1.
127. Rivaud S, Muri RM, Gaymard B, Vermersch AI, Pierrot-Deseilligny C. Eye movement disorders after frontal eye field lesions in humans. Exp Brain Res. 1994;102(1):110–20.
128. Morrow MJ, Sharpe JA. Deficits of smooth-pursuit eye movement after unilateral frontal lobe lesions. Ann Neurol. 1995;37(4):443–51.

129. Lekwuwa GU, Barnes GR. Cerebral control of eye movements. II. Timing of anticipatory eye movements, predictive pursuit and phase errors in focal cerebral lesions. Brain. 1996;119(Pt 2):491–505.
130. Braun DI, Boman DK, Hotson JR. Anticipatory smooth eye movements and predictive pursuit after unilateral lesions in human brain. Exp Brain Res. 1996;110(1):111–6.
131. Van der Stigchel S, van Koningsbruggen M, Nijboer TC, List A, Rafal RD. The role of the frontal eye fields in the oculomotor inhibition of reflexive saccades: evidence from lesion patients. Neuropsychologia. 2012;50(1):198–203.
132. Kurkin S, Takeichi N, Akao T, Sato F, Fukushima J, Kaneko CR, et al. Neurons in the caudal frontal eye fields of monkeys signal three-dimensional tracking. Ann N Y Acad Sci. 2003;1004:262–70.
133. Yang Q, Kapoula Z. Distinct control of initiation and metrics of memory-guided saccades and vergence by the FEF: a TMS study. PLoS One. 2011;6(5):e20322.
134. Vernet M, Quentin R, Chanes L, Mitsumasu A, Valero-Cabre A. Frontal eye field, where art thou? Anatomy, function, and non-invasive manipulation of frontal regions involved in eye movements and associated cognitive operations. Front Integr Neurosci. 2014;8:66.
135. Gaymard B, Pierrot-Deseilligny C, Rivaud S. Impairment of sequences of memory-guided saccades after supplementary motor area lesions. Ann Neurol. 1990;28(5):622–6.
136. Gaymard B, Rivaud S, Pierrot-Deseilligny C. Role of the left and right supplementary motor areas in memory-guided saccade sequences. Ann Neurol. 1993;34(3):404–6.
137. Berdyyeva TK, Olson CR. Intracortical microstimulation of supplementary eye field impairs ability of monkeys to make serially ordered saccades. J Neurophysiol. 2014;111(8):1529–40.
138. Husain M, Parton A, Hodgson TL, Mort D, Rees G. Self-control during response conflict by human supplementary eye field. Nat Neurosci. 2003;6(2):117–8.
139. Pierrot-Deseilligny C, Muri RM, Nyffeler T, Milea D. The role of the human dorsolateral prefrontal cortex in ocular motor behavior. Ann N Y Acad Sci. 2005;1039:239–51.
140. Pierrot-Deseilligny C, Muri RM, Rivaud-Pechoux S, Gaymard B, Ploner CJ. Cortical control of spatial memory in humans: the visuooculomotor model. Ann Neurol. 2002;52(1):10–9.
141. Pierrot-Deseilligny C, Muri RM, Ploner CJ, Gaymard B, Demeret S, Rivaud-Pechoux S. Decisional role of the dorsolateral prefrontal cortex in ocular motor behaviour. Brain. 2003;126(Pt 6):1460–73.
142. Gaymard B, Francois C, Ploner CJ, Condy C, Rivaud-Pechoux S. A direct prefrontotectal tract against distractibility in the human brain. Ann Neurol. 2003;53(4):542–5.

143. Condy C, Rivaud-Pechoux S, Ostendorf F, Ploner CJ, Gaymard B. Neural substrate of antisaccades: role of subcortical structures. Neurology. 2004;63(9):1571–8.
144. Ploner CJ, Gaymard BM, Rivaud-Pechoux S, Pierrot-Deseilligny C. The prefrontal substrate of reflexive saccade inhibition in humans. Biol Psychiatry. 2005;57(10):1159–65.
145. Gaymard B, Rivaud S, Cassarini JF, Dubard T, Rancurel G, Agid Y, et al. Effects of anterior cingulate cortex lesions on ocular saccades in humans. Exp Brain Res. 1998;120(2):173–83.
146. Phillips JM, Johnston K, Everling S. Effects of anterior cingulate microstimulation on pro- and antisaccades in nonhuman primates. J Cogn Neurosci. 2011;23(2):481–90.
147. Emeric EE, Brown JW, Leslie M, Pouget P, Stuphorn V, Schall JD. Performance monitoring local field potentials in the medial frontal cortex of primates: anterior cingulate cortex. J Neurophysiol. 2008;99(2):759–72.
148. Polli FE, Barton JJ, Cain MS, Thakkar KN, Rauch SL, Manoach DS. Rostral and dorsal anterior cingulate cortex make dissociable contributions during antisaccade error commission. Proc Natl Acad Sci U S A. 2005;102(43):15700–5.
149. Petit L, Orssaud C, Tzourio N, Salamon G, Mazoyer B, Berthoz A. PET study of voluntary saccadic eye movements in humans: basal ganglia-thalamocortical system and cingulate cortex involvement. J Neurophysiol. 1993;69(4):1009–17.
150. Anderson TJ, Jenkins IH, Brooks DJ, Hawken MB, Frackowiak RS, Kennard C. Cortical control of saccades and fixation in man. A PET study. Brain. 1994;117(Pt 5):1073–84.
151. Doricchi F, Perani D, Incoccia C, Grassi F, Cappa SF, Bettinardi V, et al. Neural control of fast-regular saccades and antisaccades: an investigation using positron emission tomography. Exp Brain Res. 1997;116(1):50–62.
152. Heide W, Binkofski F, Seitz RJ, Posse S, Nitschke MF, Freund HJ, et al. Activation of frontoparietal cortices during memorized triple-step sequences of saccadic eye movements: an fMRI study. Eur J Neurosci. 2001;13(6):1177–89.
153. Milea D, Lehericy S, Rivaud-Pechoux S, Duffau H, Lobel E, Capelle L, et al. Antisaccade deficit after anterior cingulate cortex resection. Neuroreport. 2003;14(2):283–7.

Index

A. Shaikh, F. Wang, *Eye Movements in the Critical Care Setting*,
https://doi.org/10.1007/978-3-030-70221-2